Objective Structured Medicine

Objective Structured Medicine

Kunjumon I. Vadakkan
M.B; B.S., M. D.
Licentiate of the Medical Council of Canada

iUniverse, Inc.
New York Lincoln Shanghai

Objective Structured Medicine

iUniverse books may be ordered through booksellers or by contacting:

iUniverse
2021 Pine Lake Road, Suite 100
Lincoln, NE 68512
www.iuniverse.com
1-800-Authors (1-800-288-4677)

The author has taken every effort to ensure that the information contained herein is accurate. However, due to the constantly changing nature of the medical sciences and the possibility of human error, the reader is encouraged to consult with other sources of information that may become available. While the information in this book is believed to be true and accurate at the date of going to press, the author cannot accept any legal responsibility or liability for any errors or omissions that may be made. This book contains information relating to general principles of medical examination that should not be construed as specific instructions for individual patients. Manufacturer's product information and package inserts should be reviewed for current information, including contraindications, dosages and precautions.

ISBN-13: 978-0-595-39756-3 (pbk)
ISBN-10: 0-595-39756-5 (pbk)

Printed in the United States of America

Preface to the first edition

I have great pleasure to introduce this book for medical students and residents who are preparing for various objective structured clinical examinations. I have used my experience both as a physician and as a teacher in laying out the contents. Good clinical examination need both knowledge and communication skills. Clinical skill assessment engrains both components with equal importance. In addition, physicians are often required to deliver the medical care within a fixed time. Assessment of this skill is also an important component during the examination. Therefore, the main focus of this book is to provide the candidate with a list of appropriate points required during the limited time of the examination. I warmly welcome readers who would like to participate in the next edition of this book.

I am grateful to my wife Rita and daughter Pearl for their support throughout the preparation of the manuscript. I thank iUniverse publishing team for the excellent job.

22th April, 2006   Kunjumon I. Vadakkan

Contents

How to use this book

1. Familiarize with the abbreviations as they are used almost always in clinical cases and throughout this book.

2. It is at your advantage to form study groups. Groups of 3 or 4 are found to be very efficient. Continuous feedbacks as well as willingness to accept constructive criticisms are essential elements for a successful group. Regular meetings for OSCE preparation are very essential. Read before you go for the OSCE practice sessions. Adjust time, and conduct the stations, as it is a real station. Giving 4 to 5 stations continuously to one person is found to be very successful in managing time and to get a feel of the real exam.

3. A note to the international medical graduates (IMGs): When I started my OSCE exam preparations, I was wondering how to finish both history taking and physical examination in 10 or 15 minutes. Later, I found that this time is sufficient. The main reason is that IMGs speak English slowly. Therefore practice spoken English; practice stations with your colleague. This is the most important message.

Section 1

Introduction

Objective structured clinical examinations (OSCE) are set to assess the skills of physicians objectively. Here the application of the knowledge of medicine is tested in a clinical setting is assessed. Communication skills are the paramount in assessing and delivering care in a doctor-patient relationship. It is the basis of patient agreement and compliance, patient and physician satisfaction and bilateral respect and trust. The key points to remember in such a relationship are to maintain the following patient-centered approaches. During clinical skill examinations the delivery of the clinical knowledge through proper communication skills is assessed.

- Introduce yourself. Try to use your patient's name during your introduction and then through the interview.
- Confirm with the patient any information about the case that is given before you start the station.
- Start with an open-ended question.
- Put the patient at ease during the interview.
- Maintain appropriate body posture, body language and eye contact.
- Use a professional conversational style.
- Avoid all medical jargons. Use patient's language.
- Effectively mix open and closed questions.

- Seek clarification of the patient's statements.
- Identify and understand "hidden agenda".
- Recognize and respond to patients' verbal and non verbal cues.
- Make a connection with the patient.
- Listen, don't interrupt patient's conversations.
- Interview, not interrogate.
- Express empathy, support and concern.
- Facilitate and direct an interview without controlling it.
- Respect and value the patient
- Avoid judgmental statements.
- Honesty and truth-telling: If you don't know say "I don't know".
- Cope with professional boundary issues.
- Manage hope.
- Commitment, trust and confidence. Avoid paternalism.
- Listen actively.
- Achieve a common ground with the patient.
- Level the playing field and
- Deal with both power and patient vulnerabilities.
- Seek permission and offer notification when exploring sensitive areas.
- Skills of negotiation and sharing.
- Control of one's own anger and frustration.
- Effectively bring closure to an interview.
- SP will not lie no matter how a question is asked.
- If the examiner says "no" move on to another line of questioning.
- For some cases there may be more than one issue, either a major psychosocial issue with minor medical problems (vasectomy reversal v/s midlife crisis) or a major medical problem with minor psychosocial issue (diabetic with problems at home) so don't get stuck in one aspect of the interview.
- Keep checking back with your patient to clarify mutual understanding.
- Do not make assumptions regarding marriage, relationships, children, stepchildren, work, sexuality, living arrangements etc.
- Get a picture of your patient's home and work life-support system, stresses, responsibilities, coping mechanisms (alcohol, exercise).
- Observe and acknowledge cues and clues (You seem a little anxious. Can you tell me the reason?).
- Identify the medical concerns, patient's concerns and contextual concerns and verbalize them to your patient.
- Recognize that there is a significant family problem.
- Deal with a patient suffering from multiple active problems.

- Identify patient who has had difficulty establishing effective therapeutic alliances with physicians.
- Explore patient's sexual orientation and how it is affecting his/her life situation.
- Decide on a course of action to help a patient in a difficult decision making process.
- Demonstrate tact, empathy and openness in dealing with sensitive issues.
- Engage your patient in the treatment process.
- Do not allow yourself to be judgmental of the patient, his/her opinions, ideas or situation.
- Discuss plans for any medical tests or P/Examinations—include your patient in the planning and ask about questions or concerns.
- Don't be afraid to admit if you don't know something—offer to research it.
- If things are not going too well—you've made a mistake, the interview has lost focus. Acknowledge it.
- You will be told when there are 1/2 minutes remaining. Use this time to summarize, check that you have a full account and that you and your patient understand and agree to the agenda, also ask if there are any more questions.

Stations evaluate candidates' abilities to establish effective relationships with their patients by using active communication skills. The emphasis is not to test the ability to make a medical diagnosis and then to treat it.

Patient centered conversation

- How may I help you today?
- It looks as though......
- How do you feel about this?
- Do you mind if......
- Let me make sure I've understood....
- Do you mind if we go over this?
- I understand you've come in to...and we'll get back to that but tell me a little about......
- Have you got any ideas about this?
- I can see this isn't easy for you to talk about.
- Am I the first person you have talked to about this?
- I know this isn't easy to talk about but I need to know in order to get the whole picture......
- Can you move the draw sheet little up?
- Would you like to help....quit?

- I am concerned about your smoking.
- How do you feel about it?
- What do you think is going on?
- How has it affected your life?
- I will run some tests.
- It is normal to be upset.
- It must be very hard for you.
- It seems that you are angry and anxious about it.
- I will try to make you comfortable.
- Are you aware of your HIV status?
- Give me a few minutes to ask you some questions first, and then we will come to those points (to a talkative patient).
- What are your priorities to be discussed today (if too many complaints)
- I am really concerned about your baby and I would like to encourage you to quit smoking.
- We'll see how this work, we can always readjust if we need to.
- Does this sound okay to you?
- So, I'll order these tests (say what tests and for what).....and you'll watch your diet for the next 2 weeks and we'll see how it goes, OK?
- We'll make an appointment for......we'll see you then.
- Is there anything I've missed?
- Is there anything else you'd like to talk about?

General frame for H/o taking

- Present illness—Onset, course, duration. If it is pain—PQRST (Pointation-Can you point where is the pain, Quality-What type of a pain is this, Radiation-Is it going anywhere else, Severity-On a scale of 1 to 10, 1 being the least, how do you rate this pain? Timing-What time of the day you have this pain). Get details of all expected associated symptoms. This depends on the age and sex of the patient. For females—e.g. whether pregnant or not.
- Ask whether patient has any other illnesses. Do you have any lung problems, heart problems, thyroid problems, kidney problems, liver problems, diabetes, and high blood pressure? Are you taking any medications? (Prescription, over the counter, OCPs, vitamins, herbals). Are you allergic to any medications?
- Ladies—Menstrual H/o—menarche, menopause, flow, volume, pain etc. GPAL—Gravida—Para-How many times did you become pregnant. Abortions—How many abortions (before 20 weeks of gestation) did you have? Living—How many children are alive now.

- Old age—Ask for ADL and IADL.
  ADL = Activities of daily living (DEATH)—Dressing, Eating, Ambulating, Toileting, Hygiene.
  IADL = Instrumental activities of daily life (SHAFT)—Shopping, Housekeeping, Accounting, Food preparation, Transportation
- Old age—polypharmacy-too many over the counter medications.
- Teenager—HEEADSS interview.
  Home—With whom are you living? Relationships, recent moves, ever run away?
  Education—attendance, grades, future plans?
  Eating—habits, anemia, obesity.
  Activities—extracurricular, best friend, social events, gangs.
  Drugs—alcohol, tobacco, with friends/alone?
  Sex—dating, orientation, experiences, contraception, pregnancies, STDs, sexual abuse
  Suicide—self esteem thoughts, plan, message, attempts, and depression.
- Past illness—Were you suffering from any health problems before? (If patient ask "like what", then ask specifically as in the previous paragraph). Were there any surgeries.
- Personal H/o—SADS HOT DOGS—smoking, alcohol, drugs, sex, hobbies, occupation, travel, diet.
- Family H/o.
- There are some musts that we need to ask for each department.

Surgery—AMPLE—allergy, medications, pregnancy, previous surgeries, last meal, last tetanus shot, events before injury
OBG—LMP, EDC, contraction, passage of blood, discharge, fetal movements
Psychiatry—stressors, delutions, hallucinations, suicidal tendencies, homicidal plans, weapon possession. Ask 3 direct questions—have you ever had depression, mania or schizophrenia, have you ever visited a psychiatrist, have you ever been treated for any mental illness, search for any systemic diseases causing psychiatric symptoms, drug use
Cardiology—risk factors, DVT, last ECG, B.P

- The ending of the station needs EPPQ(2)
  Explain what the patient is having—I think you are suffering from.....
  Plan—You can go home with medications/follow up visit/I would like to admit you in the hospital
  Prognosis—You are going to be alright. You have come to the best place for treatment. If survival is very slim—"You are seriously ill. Everything will be

done to help you". Patient should be given chance to express his views or last wishes.

Questions (2)—Is this plan OK for you? Do you have any questions?

- Other important tasks that are expected from the candidates (**CANADA**)

1. Inform the ministry of transportation (MOT) (In severe visual problems, epilepsy and any medical conditions that disables the patient to drive).
2. Form or certify the patient if the patient is going to hurt themselves or others. (Sign form 1 and give the copy (form 42) to the patient. This will give the power for the police to restrain the patient during the 7 days following-if the patient run out of the hospital). Form 1 give the opportunity to observe the patient in a hospital set up for 72 hours.

- Conditions that are likely to forget

1. Cystic fibrosis—both in respiratory and GI problems up to age 40
2. Schizophrenia
3. Head injuries (H/o)
4. Inflammatory bowel disease
5. Camera test (any H/o of scopies)

General communication skills

The following are the 4 main areas where the candidates will be evaluated.

- **Empathy** (Not sympathy)—I understand you have severe pain/I understand that it is very difficult for you.
- **Coherence** (Don't break the patient while talking)—Co-hear = Hear together.
- **Verbal**—Good spoken English ability
- **Non-verbal**—your body language—posture e.g. leaning forward shows interest, nodding your head shows you understand, talking with your hands will facilitate communication.

- After the examination cover up the patient properly
- Look at the face while palpating
- Offer medications for pain
- Don't talk during labor pain/renal colic pain
- Warm your hands and stethoscope

- Offer brochures
- Keep silence when the patient cry
- Offer napkins when the patient cry
- Always keep spousal abuse and child abuse in mind. This happens especially if the child comes with excessive crying or vomiting; but on H/o nothing positive turns out. Females coming with headache, abdominal pain and pelvic without any relevant features. Watch their body language.

Important things

- Read the task whether it is H/o only, H/o and P/E or P/E only. Do only what is asked for.
- Prepare the DDx before entering the room and ask questions for that.
- Remember, if you get the diagnosis during the initial questions, you are likely to fail in the exam. This is because your exam mark is based on your questions in the check list and not for getting the diagnosis. So even if you get the diagnosis ask all questions for your DDx. Don't let your good abilities hurt you in OSCE.
- Time management is very important. Go little fast. Never stay on one point even if the patient tries to distract you.
- Forget the station that you have just finished.

<u>Counseling—what is it?</u>

In an ideal counseling set up consist of:
Introduction
Understanding the problem
Assessing the person's knowledge and thoughts about the situation, any previous attempts to change, reasons for failure, motivation, support groups, depression and hope, and the person's idea of changing the situation.

Giving information in small chunks, communicate in person's own language.
Test whether the person understands what you are telling him by asking the question "Do you understand?" at least few times during the session.
Giving options see which plan works for him better; give time to think about the options. Give time to talk to friends, family members or members of groups that suffer the same problems and recovered.
Asking to summarize.
Asking whether s/he has any questions, give another appointment to follow up.
Referring if needed, offer support, be realistic.

Congratulating the patient for the session.

Duration and diagnosis

Psychiatry: always ask the duration, since most of the diagnosis depends on the duration of the symptoms.

Mania—7 days
Hypomania—4 days
Depression—2 weeks
Bereavement—2 months
OCD—6 months
Schizophrenia—6 months
Schizophreniform disorder—less than 6 months
Brief psychotic disorder—less than 1 month
Anorexia—less than 15% of the expected weight.

Medications—a quick review

Community acquired pneumonia-Clarithromycin 500 mgm po bid x 14 days

Peptic ulcer disease-Lansoprazole 30mg po bd-Clarithromycin 500 mg po bid-amoxycillin 1gm po bid x 7days only (HP-PAC 7 blister card pack)

Gonorrhea and Chlamydia—Cefixime 400 mg po single dose+azithromycin 1gm po single dose (All are treated with 2 single doses!!!!)

Herpes—acyclovir 400 mg po tid x 7 days.

Periodic health examination

The policies changes from country to country, state to state and time to time. However, the following is a common approach that can be used.

General
Dental hygiene
Noise control and hearing protection
Smoking cessation
Nicotine replacement

Pediatrics
Repeated exam of hips, eyes, hearing (1st year)
Routine immunizations
Hepatitis B immunization
Varicella vaccine (1-12)

Adults
Hemoccult (>50)
Sigmoidoscopy (>50) B
If Diastolic BP >90 Rx (21-64)
Follow up on caregiver concern of cognitive impairment
Multi-disciplinary post-fall assessment

Woman
Breast exam (50-69)
Mammography (50-69)
Pap smear (18-69) B
Folic acid to females of child bearing age

Special cases
Diabetes—Urine dipstick
TB high risks—Mantoux testing/INH prophylaxis to household contacts
STD high risks—voluntary HIV and gonorrhea testing
Influenza Amantidine for those exposed to index case
Immunocompetent and institutionalized->55—pneumococcal vaccination

Referal services that are often made for the patients

In addition to the medical and surgical specialities, the following refer specialists are often required in patient management.

Dietician,
Speech pathologist,
Physiotherapist,
Optometrist,
Family counselor

Section 2

Check list and instructions to standardized patients

You might have acquired a vast amount of knowledge in one or more subjects while completing your previous training. This will make you do both history taking and physical examination in more detail. Time is restricted and therefore your objective should be to complete the tasks that are listed in the check list and not to do a detailed examination. You will not be given credit for doing what is not listed in the check list.

These sections will give examples of a check list and the method of scoring.

In addition, it takes lot of time and effort to train a standardized patient (SP) by the examination board. This is to make sure that the SP interacts with the candidate only as requested by the instructions. Therefore, it is better to know samples of instructions usually given to SPs. This is facilitate your perception of the examination process and improve your scores

Instructions to SPs and check list of the station

These two areas were always kept hidden from the candidates so far. But here I present sample instructions to the SP. SPs are trained to act for a station. Usually they keep doing the same station over years. Therefore, they know how to act well for that particular station. Here is a sample station that requires high amount of skills to be an S.P and all the instructions to the SP are also given.

Question: Mr.X came to your office to know the results of the HIV test. You were on vacation when Mr.X came to your clinic last month. Your colleague Dr. Y examined Mrs.X and ordered for an HIV test. Mr.X does not want his wife to know his HIV status if it comes out to be positive. Talk to Mr.X in 10 minutes.

Fact: Mr.X is married and his wife Mrs.X is also your patient. She has an appointment with you after 4 days. Mr. X had unprotected sex in a group sex club 3 years ago for a few months before his marriage to Mr.X.

Instructions to standardized patients:

- Your name is Mr.X. Your age is 34. You are a senior clerk in a post office.
- Your job is going very well. You are happily married for the last 2.5 years to Mrs.X, an office assistant in downtown.
- You had a couple of girl friends before. But never had sex with them. 3 years ago you met with a friend who introduced you to a group sex club where you had unprotected sex with both men and ladies for most of the days for one month while you were on a trip to a foreign country.
- Your marriage to Mrs.X has been a good one.
- You have never experienced any symptoms of AIDS (e.g. weight loss, infections, night sweats, diarrhea etc.)
- You are planning to have a child with your wife. But you have a suspicion that you may have an HIV infection. You talked about it to Dr.Y during your last visit. He ordered an HIV test.
- Dr. Y had a brief conversation with you during that visit. Since you never had any symptoms of AIDS so far, you and Dr. Y were hoping for the best.
- You called the nurse in the office today morning and found that the results have come. But the nurse refused to give the results over the phone. You could not arrange an appointment for today as the day was fully booked. You are anxious to get the results and waiting in the clinic for the last one hour to get an appointment.

- *Prompt 1. (Prompts give every candidate an opportunity to face appropriate issues).*
  "What is the result doctor?"
  Doctor tells you the results after taking some time and making sure that you are ready to accept any type of an answer.
  "Are you absolutely sure". "Couldn't there be some mistake?"
- *Prompt.* "So I am going to die doctor"
  "I have AIDS and I am going to die". You become little agitated and panic.
- *Prompt 3.* "Does my wife have to know about this?"
- If the candidate (examinee) advises you to tell your wife about it you may say like this "How can I tell here this? She does not know anything about my previous sexual experiences. I can't do this". "I really love her and I can't hurt her feelings. If she finds this out, she will be devastated and I will be destroying her life. Why should we do this to her?"................. (silence).........."That will be the end of it. She will leave me. I don't want to lose her"
- *Prompt 4.* "Why does my wife have to know about this? "Why can't this information be confidential between me and you"
- "You won't tell her behind my back. Will you?"
- *Prompt 5..* "My wife is coming to you after few days. I don't want you to tell her about it"
- Mood becomes sad and hopeless
- Never agree to the doctor's idea to tell to your wife.
- *Prompt 6.* "What will you do if I don't tell her?"

Checklist for this station:
HIV and Ethics—Case 4
1. Assure that HIV test +ive does not mean that the patient has AIDS.
2. Prognosis is variable.
3. His wife should know and she has the right to know.
4. Use safe sex with your wife or other partners to prevent transmission of HIV.
5. Offer help to tell his wife.
6. Tell that wife will know that some one with whom she had sex has HIV test positive.
7. Offer follow up visit and support.

Note: This station will be used to test your communication skills and also your abilities to manage ethical issues in medical practice.

Other examples of prompts that the SPs are asked to give you

- "I want to be taken off this respirator"
- "It is my life. So I have the right to decide what to do with it"
- "What happens next?"
- "I don't want any operation"
- "It is my decision. Can you do anything without my consent?"
- "Are you going to do the surgery?"
- "Why won't you do this for me?"
- "I know my husband has cancer. I don't want you to tell him about it"
- If the candidate refuses to write a note to excuse you from an exam that your have tomorrow ask him "Why are you not writing a letter". "Why is it wrong?"
- When the candidate asks you "So you want me to tell the patient a lie?", answer back "No. I don't want you to lie to him. I am asking not to tell".
- Show anger to the candidate
- Cry now. Take napkins if the candidate offers and say thanks
- Walk out of the examination room at 7 minutes (in a 10 minute station)—Mania
- Listen to the voices that you are hearing—Schizophrenia.

SPs get very strict orders. Therefore, they will stick to that. Examples-

- If candidate does not mention about organ donation, do not use any further prompts.
- If candidate asks about organ donation, you can agree to it.
- Do not give any hint/prompt for questions from the candidate like "Do you want to discuss anything else today?"

Section 3

Medicine

Migratory arthritis
Hypertension
Fatigue
Impotence
Cardiology P/E
Diabetes counseling
Diabetic ketoacidosis
Bleeding disorder
Volume status
Counselling for high cholesterol
Counselling to quit smoking
Counseling obesity
Lymph node enlargement
Presbycusis
Torticollis

Cough

Case 1: 50 year old man comes to your office because of a chronic cough.
Case 2: 30 year old man comes to your office 24 hr after being discharged from ER because of an asthma attack. You are asked to review her condition.

O—When did you start coughing? Establish if it is chronic (> 3 weeks) or not. When was your first attack? Did the onset was gradual/sudden?
C—Is it getting worse? Is it a paroxysmal cough? Day/night? Get worse at night?
D—Do you cough every day? Again make sure that it is chronic

1. Is it a dry cough? Have you had any sputum (phlegm)? If present, ask color (changes since it started), odor, consistency and amount.
2. Aggravating factors: Exposure to smoke, pets, exercise, outside/inside home, certain areas, medications.
3. Relieving factors: Medications if any, positions.
4. Asthma: wheezing, chest tightness, gets worse at night.
5. COPD: abundant sputum in the morning easily catches a cold, SOB, signs of RHF.
6. GER: gets worse after eating, lying down, ear pain, hoarseness, wheezing.
7. TB/HIV (chronic infections): weight loss, lymphadenopathy, hemoptysis, fever, skin lesions, anorexia.
8. Postnasal drip/sinusitis: Cold symptoms before the cough started, tenderness in the face, nasal drip, halitosis, fever, previous episodes, known allergies, vasomotor rhinitis.
9. Malignancies: weight loss, hemoptysis, CP, SOB, bone pain, adenopathies.
10. ILD/collagen diseases: clubbing, fever, joint pain, eye symptoms, rash.
11. PMH: During childhood: Asthma, CF, pneumonias, allergies.
    During adulthood: UTRI, sinusitis, rhinitis, lung, heart problems, heartburn, PUD.
12. Ask about the last chest-x-ray taken.
13. Medications (ACE-I, ECASA), allergies
14. Smoking or second hand smoking, alcohol, drugs, RF, HIV, contact with people coughing, recent travels, immigrations from endemic countries. TB, previous BCG.
15. Occupation (how this interferes with your daily activities?) hobbies.
16. Family situation, family H/o.
17. D/d: a. Pneumonia b. Bronchitis c. Tuberculosis d. Asthma e. Post-nasal drip f. Tobacco addiction.
18. DWU—Chest X-ray/CBC/Tuberculin skin test (PPD)/sputum Gram's stain/pulse oximetry.

Dyspnoea

Case: 65 years old with known COPD is brought by paramedics to ER because of worsening SOB. Take the H/o.

Before starting the H/o, make sure that the patient is not in acute distress.
H/o: Analyze dyspnea:
O—sudden/gradual onset? When was the first attack? At rest/during exercise?
C—Persistent or intermittent? How frequent? Is it getting worse?
D—How long does the episode(s) last? Did you get any treatment? Did it work?

1. Assessment of severity: Ask particular situation such as: SOB when walking, climbing stairs, minimal activities (ADL/IADL), at rest and talking.
2. Aggravating factors: worsening on exertion, emotion, positions, smoking, pets, cold, new meds (beta blockers).
3. Alleviating factors: Medications. Recent increase or decrease in dose of medications.
4. If known COPD/asthmatic, ask: Hospitalizations, intubations, CPAP treatment, pneumothorax.
5. Associated symptoms: cough, wheezing, fever, chills, hemoptysis, CP, fatigue, hoarseness, paraneoplastic symptoms, CHF: orthopnea (how many pillows?), nocturia, PND, leg edema, anorexia.
6. PMH: lung, heart, TB contacts, DVT, DM, PUD, asthma, pneumonias, kidney.
7. Medications (steroids, puffers.), allergies
8. Smoking, alcohol, drugs, HIV status, travel, occupation, diet, family situation
9. Family H/o.

If you have to examine the patient

1. General inspection: Ask the vitals if not given: Is the patient in respiratory distress? Posture, tripod position, accessory muscles, intercostal retraction, tracheal tub, difficulty speaking, paradoxical movement of the abdomen. LOC: somnolence, alert, confused?
2. Inspection of the face: Horner's syndrome, central cyanosis, pursed lip breathing, plethora.
3. Inspection of the hands: peripheral cyanosis, clubbing, nicotine stains, wasting muscles, asterixis, tremor (beta agonist or hypercapnia).
4   Palpation; Midline trachea, LNs.

5. Chest:
   Inspection: shape, barrel, intercostal retraction, scars, dilated veins.
   Palpation: trachea displaced, heave, respiratory expansion, tactile vocal fremitus
   Percussion: dull/hyper-resonant; apices of lungs, ant-post, upper, lower, middle lobes, diaphragmatic excursion, upper border of liver.
   Auscultation: air entry, strider, vesicular breathing, added sounds (crackles, wheezing,) pleural rub.
6. Leg edemas, CVS signs of cor pulmonale, JVP, liver size.
7. Special tests:
a. Using the ulnar aspect of the palm—do tactile fremitus (Ask patient say 99)
b. Normal breathing sound is vesicular.
c. Bronchial breathing is normally heard over the manubrium. It is also heard in consolidation in pneumonia.
d. Using the stethoscope hear the sound over the lungs when patient says 99. Normally it is not heard as 99—No bronchophony.
e. Using the stethoscope hear the sound when patient whisper 99. Normally not heard as 99—No whispering pectoriloqy.
f. Using the stethoscope hear the sound when patient says "ee". Normally not heard as "ee"—No egophony.
g. Forced expiratory time: Exhales completely in <3 sec: COPD >4 sec

8. D/d: 1.Pneumothorax 2.Pulmonary embolus 3.Pneumonia
9. DWU: CXR/Pulse oximetry or ABG/Spiral CT scan or V/Q scan, bilateral lower limb venous Doppler.

Headache

Case 1: 45 year old man in ER C/o of headaches and vomiting for 1 month.
Case 2: 26 year old woman in ER complaining of worsening of a new headache.
Case 3: 50 year old man in ER because of headache and vomiting for a few hrs.
Case 4: 20 year old female is brought by her mother to ER because of headaches and fever.
Case 5: 68 year old woman in your office complaining of right side headache.

Make sure that the patient is stable.
If the patient is very sick, start with the ABCs (e. g: SAH or meningitis).
If the patient is in pain reassure the patient saying that you will give pain killers after the examination and begin taking the H/o.

O-Sudden/gradual? When did the pain start?
C-Paroxismal? In clusters? On-off, wax-wane, steady?
D-Is this for the first time? Had it affected you before? How long was an attack? Is this attack different from usual ones? Previous ER visits.
Analyze the pain:
P-Uni/bilateral. Make sure if this is a headache or the pain is in the face (nose, teeth, throat, ears, and neck).
Q-Dull, throbbing, sharp, tension, "The worse pain of my life" (SAH)
R-Where is the pain going?
S-Scale 1-10,
T-Morning—ICH; Evening—tension headache; No-timing—migraine.

1. Make sure that it is not associated with trauma
2. Trigger factors: exercise, glare (driving)/light, noise, hunger/thirst, stressful situations, food (alcohol), cough/sneezing, chewing, combing hair, menses, medications.
3. Is it getting worse? Does the pain wake you at night? Prevent you to go to work? Doing your daily activities?
4. Threshold factors: depressed mood, disturbance in sleep, menses, BCP, HRT.
5. Relieving factors: lying down, medications, darkness, quiet room.
6. Red flags in headaches
7. Associated symptoms:
   Brain mass: vomiting, weakness, seizures, decreased vision, LOC, decreased hearing, tinnitus, vertigo, gait instability, change in personality, SOB,
   Meningitis: fever, decreased consciousness, neck stiffness, rash, N/V.

SAH: neck stiffness, decreased consciousness, N/V.

Temporal arteritis: scalp pain, decreased vision, problems chewing, fatigue, muscle pain, fever,

Glaucoma: eye pain, decreased vision, N/Vomiting.

Migraine: visual/auditory/olfactory hallucinations, opthalmoplegia, numbness, N/V.

Cluster headaches: tears, red eye, running nose.

Systemic conditions: CP, SOB, HTN (encephalopathy), edemas (renal failure),

PMH: HTN, DM, trauma, neurological diseases, psychiatric diseases, CTD, sinusitis, otitis, trigeminal neuralgia,

8.   Medications: BCP, antibiotics, vitamins, steroids (cerebral pseudo-tumor), allergies.

9.   Social: Occupation, HIV status, smoking, alcohol, drugs, interference with daily activities,

10. Family H/o: brain tumors, migraine, strokes, other cancers.

11. Common migraine—no aura/classical has aura: Both unilateral throbbing. Photo and phonophobia. Rx—analgesics, neuroleptics, vasoactive medications.

12. Tension headache—never during sleep—posterior and occipital/increase with stressors. Increased ICP—worse in the morning or bending down Rx—CT

13. Temporal arteritis-scalp tenderness-jaw claudication/visual disturbances.

1) Brain tumor 2) "New onset of pain becoming worse" due to OCP. Rx: Stop pills 3) SAH 4) Meningitis 5) Temporal arteritis.

Case 7: 50 yr old woman with headache and normal vitals. Take H/o.
Describe appropriate investigations and treatment for temporal arteritis.

1.   Polymyalgia rheumatica (most likely from the question).Unilateral lancinating pain with swelling and tenderness in the temporal area.

2.   It is related to temporal arteritis and may a systemic variant of the same disease.

3.   Both have low grade fever, malaise, anorexia, weight loss, bilateral proximal muscle weakness, aching and pain and joint inflammation.

4.   Jaw claudication, stroke and blindness may occur due to vasculitic occlusion of arterial supply.

5. Investigations: CBC (mild anaemia with increased WBC), ESR (>50 mm/hr, normal 30), C-reactive protein, liver enzymes, temporal artery biopsy.

6. Treatment: In the absence of visual symptoms, without waiting for biopsy, start high dose oral prednisone, 60 mg OD until symptoms subside and ESR normal, then 40 mg OD for 4-6 weeks, then taper to 5-10 mg OD for 2 yrs. (Relapses occur in 50% if treatment is terminated before 2 yrs).

7. Treatment does not alter biopsy results if the sample is taken within 2 weeks. Monitor ESR regularly.

8. If visual symptoms are present, or develop during treatment, the patient is admitted and given IV prednisone 1 g q 12 hr for 5 days.

9. D/d: a. Brain tumor b. OCP induced c. SAH d. Meningitis e. Temporal arteritis
    f. Subdural hematoma g. Tension headache h. Migraine headache

10. DWU: CT scan of the head

Seizures

Case 1: 30 year old man conies to your office complaining of spells.
Case 2: 50 year old non epileptic woman comes to ER after she had a seizure episode.
Case 3: 75 year old man is brought by paramedics after having seizures and post-ictal right side weakness.

To make sure you check your ABCs before taking the H/o
Ask what does the patient mean by spells? (seizure, convulsion, fainting, dizziness, "feel fanny".
O-When, how did it start? What were you doing when it start?
C-Paroxysmal episodes? How many attacks have you had?
D-How long is an attack? Previous hospitalizations?

1. Analyze the seizure (witness).
2. Aura (N/V, flashing lights, dizziness, odors, déjà vu), body position, color of skin.
3. During: LOC, falls down, eye twitching, neck turning, cyanosis, tongue biting, urinary incontinence, lip smacking, automatic movements.
4. After: Injuries in the head? Confusion, myalgia, amnesia, weakness, cyanosis, respiratory difficulty.
5. Precipitating factors: Make sure that is not associated to trauma, fever, alcohol, drugs, medications, stress, computer/TV, infections and tiredness.
6. Behavior change, irritability, memory/concentration problems and accidents.
7. Problems learning, performing activities and holding conversations?
8. Amnesia: have you found yourself wandering in a new place?
9. Brain occupying lesions: weakness, decreased vision, headaches.
10. Metastasis: if primary known: lung/breast/prostate/colon/melanoma.
11. PMH: Head trauma, DM, HTN, epilepsy, meningitis during childhood, cancer, strokes, bleeding tendency, leukemias, lymphomas.
12. Medications: If the patient is epileptic make sure that she is taking the correct doses, interactions with other drugs.
13. Allergies.
14. Social: Occupation, smoking, alcohol, drugs, impact in daily activities.
15. Driving: Ask license even if not driving at the moment but the patient has a license you have to report it to the MOT.
16. Family support, finances, drug plan, hobbies.
17. Family H/o: brain tumors, cancer, epilepsy, related conditions.

18. Explain to the patient that until the final Dx is made, his/her driver's license is going to be suspended. S/he will be contacted by the MOT.

1: Partial focal seizure; 2: Brain tumor; 3: Stroke

a) If seizure free from 12 month on medication—can drive a private vehicle (Canada).
b) If seizure is absent for 5 yrs on medication—can drive a public vehicle (Canada).

Case 4: 16 yr old known epileptic on Dilantin (phenytoin), is having 3 seizures per month and requests better medication. Manage. (Findings: not taking medications, experiencing stress).

1. Describe seizures, frequency, duration, what body parts affected and in what order, premonitory signs, post-ictal state (decrease in level of consciousness, headache, sensory phenomena), degree of control achieved with Dilantin at what dose and for how long? Age of first seizure.
2. Side effects of Dilantin: Drowsiness, poor concentration, poor performance in school, acne, nystagmus, dysarthria, ataxias, peripheral neuropathy, hypertrichosis (excessive hairiness), gingival hypertrophy.
3. Number and description of recent seizures, are they different from previous seizures? Is the patient having any new symptoms such as headache, morning vomiting, new neurological deficits?
4. If the drug has worked in the past, why does the patient believe it is no longer effective?
5. Compliance: Is the patient taking meds? Why not? Problems at school or at home?
6. Ask about relationship problems.
7. Depression screen. Social supports, medications, drugs and alcohol, smoking, allergies, PMH, family H/o, ROS.
8. P/E: Neurologic exam including MMSE, cranial nerves, bulk, tone, power, sensation, cerebellar exam, deep tendon reflexes.
9. Send blood for serum Dilantin level.
10. Management: Discuss importance of compliance.
11. Chronic alcohol intake may decrease blood levels of Phenytoin.
12. Acute alcohol intake, sedatives, cocaine, amphetamines, and insulin can precipitate seizures.
13. Fatigue can lower seizure threshold.
14. If patient has anxiety or stress, s/he may need counselling.

15. If patient has severe side effects or poor seizure control with dilantin, a second drug may be added (usually carbamazepine or valproic acid).
16. Discuss to avoid driving.
17. Inform the MOT of the patient's seizure disorder.
18. Discuss what to do in the event of a seizure. Do not insert objects into the patient's mouth. Turn the patient on his/her side while seizing.
19. Call ambulance if seizure doesn't stop in 10 min.
20. Arrange regular follow-up and check serum Dilantin levels.

Case 5: 16 yr old boy with epilepsy documented by neurologist, comes to you because he does not want to see his parent's family doctor. Wants a driver's licence. Take H/o and counsel.

1. Outline a treatment plan consisting of EEG, CT head, metabolic screen, medications (if not done already).
2. Follow up appointments.
3. Get the parents involved if possible.
4. Arrange regular follow up to monitor progress and serum anti-epileptic levels.

Pneumonia

Case 1: 30 year old man with a fever and cough for 3 days.
Case 2: Known HIV positive patient comes with fever and cough for 3 weeks.
Case 3: 60 year old man with known COPD complains of fever and increase in cough.

1. OCD: establish sudden/insidious onset.
2. Sputum (phlegm)—color, amount, odor, consistency.
3. Fever: pattern, chills.
4. Associated symptoms: SOB, CP, wheezing, hemoptysis, diarrhea, night sweats, rash, previous UTRI, earache, weight loss, hoarseness, joint pain, eye symptoms, headache, adenopathies.
5. PMH: Asthma, heart disease, TB, COPD, compliance to medications, cancers. (leukemias, lymphomas) chemotherapy leading to neutropenia.
6. Hospitalizations, surgeries (splenectomy).
7. Flu shot, allergies, medications, prophylaxis.
8. Occupation, recent travels, TB exposure, contact with sick people, pets.
9. Flu shot, RF, HIV
10. Family H/o.

When you have a Dx of pneumonia examine if
1. Is it a community acquired or hospital acquired?
2. Is this an immunocompromised patient (HIV, COPD, DM, CHF, CRF, cancer) or not? If yes, is s/he neutropenic or not? Febrile neutropenia is an emergency in infectious diseases.
3. Rx for community acquired pneumonia: Clarithromycin 500mgm bd PO x 14 days

Cases:
1: Streptococcus pneumonia
2: PCP
3: Pneumonia in COPD (Bugs: H. Influenza, Moraxella, Klebsiella, E.Coli, Legionella.

Case4: 65 yr old male outpatient with SOB, cough, sputum. Take H/o and perform a P/E. Findings: Lobar consolidation with yellow-green sputum. Given a diagnosis of pneumonia, recommend treatment.

1. H/o: Cough, sputum (colour), fever, chills, malaise, fatigue, SOB, increase in asthmatic symptoms (wheeze, cough), preceding viral illness.
2. Onset, chronology of symptoms, positional factors (orthopnea), chest pain, ankle swelling.
3. H/o of COPD?
4. Medications, compliance with meds (use of puffers), drugs of abuse (alcohol), smoking, allergies, PMH, family H/o, ROS.
5. P/E: Both cardiology and respiratory.
6. For diagnosis of community-acquired pneumonia, admit if patient is systemically ill (may have septicaemia).
7. If the patient is debilitated, or hypoxia is a feature (send blood cultures and give oxygen).

Case5: HIV positive man. 1 week of shortness of breath, cough, fatigue. Perform a P/E. Give DDx for a CXR showing a fine reticular pattern in the left lower lobe. Manage.

1. Respiratory examination.
2. Pulmonary effusion decreases transmission of vocal sounds to the chest wall, while consolidation (in pneumonia) increases it.
3. Signs of consolidation: Percussion dullness, crackles, bronchial breath sounds, increased tactile fremitus, increased voice transmission (bronchophony, egophony, whispered petroliloquy).
4. Signs of HIV infection (and possible AIDS): Check skin for Kaposi's sarcoma, pharynx for thrush or hairy leukoplakia, palpate neck, clavicle, axilla and groin for lymph nodes enlargement due to non-Hodgkin's lymphoma, examine abdomen for hepatic and splenic enlargement.
5. D/d of unilateral lobar reticular pattern on CXR: Pneumocystis carinii pneumonia (PCP), cytomegalovirus (CMV), tuberculosis, cryptococcus neoformans, hemophilus, streptococcus, mycoplasma and chlamydia.
6. The classic CXR of PCP, an AIDS-defining illness is bilateral hilar infiltrates but X-ray findings are variable and may be alveolar or interstitial.
7. Investigations: O_2 sat. ABG, CBC with differential and CD4 count, LDH (elevated in 95% of PCP pneumonias and not in other pneumonias), blood cultures, sputum for cytology, gram stain, culture and TB stain if sputum available (cough usually non-productive and may fail to induce sputum), bronchoscopy with cytology, gram stain and culture of bronchial washings and brushings.
8. Treatment: DS Septran 2 tabs QID x 14 days outpatient with 1 tab OD or BID 3/week continued as prophylaxis.

9. In severe illness, admit to hospital, give IV Septran at same dose and prednisone 40 mg BID x 5 days, then 20 mg OD for prophylaxis.
10. Counselling and referral to support organization. Follow-up appointment.

Sudden loss of vision

Case 1: 50 year old diabetic patient in ER complaining of one side blindness.
Case 2: 62 year old man comes to ER complaining of right side blindness.
Case 3: 35 year old woman comes to ER because of right side eye pain and new onset of blindness.

1.   Make sure that it is blindness and not diplopia/ptosis.
2.   Ask about visual acuity. No light at all? No objects at all?
O—Sudden/gradual? Uni/bilateral? Recurrent? Partial/total?
C—On/off? Transient/persistent?
D—Minutes/hours/days? first time? previous hospitalizations?

3.   Retinal detachment: Floaters, like curtains coming down? painless?
4.   TIA: Paresthesia, weakness, headaches, painless.
5.   MS: Pain, paresthesia, weakness, facial palsy, urinary incontinence.
6.   Temporal arteritis: Unilateral scalp tenderness, jaw claudication, fever.
7.   Migraine: Headaches, photophobia. N/V, light flashing, aura.
8.   HTN retinopathy: Headaches, partial field defect.
9.   Macular degeneration: Painless, ongoing, partial loss of vision (partial visual defect)
10. HIV—related: Toxoplasmosis, CMV.
11. Gaucoma: Pain, progressive decrease in V/A, not sudden LOV.
12. Hyperviscosity syndrome: Multiple myeloma, Waldenstrom, CML.
13. Conversion disorder: No anatomical lesion found, la bella indifference.
14. PMH: HTN, DM, eye diseases, migraine, MS, strokes, valvular heart diseases (AF).
15. Medications, allergies.
16. Social: Occupation. HIV, alcohol, smoking, drugs.
17. Family H/o: HTN, DM, strokes.
18. This is an emergency. So you have to admit the patient and do the proper referral.
19. While wailing the final treatment can start anticoagulation, IV steroids, anti-HTN.

Cases: 1. Retinal detachment 2. TIA 3.MS (optic neuritis)

Dizziness

Case 1: 32 years old woman comes to ER complaining of dizziness.
Case 2: 46 yrs old man in your office complaining of hearing loss and dizziness.
Case 3: 68 years old woman is brought to ER by paramedics because of acute onset of dizziness, vomiting and fall.

2 types: 1) Vertigo is vestibular 2) Non-vertiginous is non-vestibular.

Vestibular (Vertigo)

2 types based on the feeling.
a) Objective (external world seems to resolve around)
b) Subjective (individual revolves in space)

2 types based on the etiology.
a) Central (15%)—brain stem, cerebellar—tumor, stroke, drugs, M.S
b) Peripheral (85%)—inner ear, VIII nerve—idiopathic (Miniere's, BPV), tumour, trauma, drugs, infection.

Non-vestibular (Non-vertigo)

Feel light-headed, giddy, dazed, mentally confused, disoriented.
3 types
1) Vascular: VBI, basilar migraine, TIA, orthostatic hypotension, Stokes Adams, arrhythmia—CHF, AS, vasovagal episode.
2) Ocular—decreased visual acuity.
3) Psychogenic—diagnosis of exclusion.

1. Make sure that the patient is stable and can cooperate with you in the H/o.
2. Make sure what the patient means by "dizziness"?
3. Is it vertigo: Things spin around you?
4. Is it lightheadedness: Fanny in my head?
5. Is it unsteadiness: Trouble walking or keeping balance?
6. Is it syncope or near fainting? Transitory LOC? Did you feel that you were going to pass out?
7. Is it lateralizing? Do you feel like going to fall on one side?
O—Sudden/gradual? What where you doing when this sensation start?
C—Steady course or paroxysmal? In attacks? On-off? Wax-wane?
D—First time? Did this happen before? Any hospitalizations?

8. How long is an attack: Seconds-BPV/minutes—Meniere's/days—VIII neuronitis/weeks—acoustic neurinoma. (More the time, more severe it is).
9. Precipitating factors: Position of head (lying), rolling, stress, URTI, ear infection.
10. Relieving factors: Closing the eyes, resting still, meds.
11. BPV: N/V, vertigo, imbalance if standing, trouble reading the newspaper.
12. Neuronitis: N/V, imbalance, vertigo, hearing impairment.
13. Meniere's: N/V, vertigo, hearing loss, fullness in the ear.
14. Neurinoma: Hearing loss, tinnitus, lateralization, imbalance, and nistagmus.
15. Cerebellar disease: N/V, weakness, ataxia, dysarthria, nistagmus.
16. Other causes: Tremor, diplopia, seizures, sweating, hunger.
17. PMH: Head trauma, HTN, DM, ear diseases, epilepsy, anemia, URTI, heart disease, depression, BPV, brain tumor.
18. Medications: Anti-HTN, ASA, antiepileptic (hydantoin intoxication), diuretics, sedatives, antibiotics.
19. Allergies.
20. Social: Smoking, alcohol, drugs, HIV, sex, occupation, impact in everyday life.
21. Able to work? drive? read?
22. Family H/o.
23. Investigations: Cardiac, neurologic, vascular, peripheral exams
24. ECG, EEG, 24 hr Holter monitor, treadmill test, carotid and vestibular Doppler, ENT, audiometry, MRI, 3 min hyperventilation trial.

When you finish your interview think if,
1) Is this vertigo?
2) If vertigo, is it central or peripheral?
3) How would you study this patient? Do you have to admit him/her?
4) Possible treatments
5) Prognosis.

Cases:
1. BPV 2. Acoustic neurinoma. 3.Cerebellar infarction.
Case 4: Elderly lady with syncopeal attacks. Take a H/o. Give a DDx. What investigations would you order?

1. H/o: Onset, chronology, description of events.
2. Have the patient's episodes been witnessed?

3. Does the patient lose consciousness, are there warning signs pr post-ictal symptoms, can the patient prevent episode by sitting down or by other means?

4. If dizziness is a feature, is this light-headedness or true vertigo (vertigo means that the patient senses actual movement of either the room of themselves).

5. Associated fatigue, weakness, nausea, vomiting, chest pain, SOB, palpitations, focal neurological symptoms.

6. PMH (DM, heart disease), medications, drug use, alcohol, smoking, allergies, family H/o, ROS.

7. DDx: Medication induced: digoxin (bradycardia), lasix (hypovolemia). Cardiovascular: arrhythmia, valvular disease, subclavian steal.

8. Metabolic: Hypoglycemia.

9. CNS: Seizures (narcolepsy, tumour), stroke/TIA, cervical spondylosis.

10. Anxiety with hyperventilation.

11. Middle ear (BPV, acoustic neuroma, Meniere's disease).

12. Autonomic: Vagal, orthostatic hypotension.

13. Digoxin overdose: Anorexia, nausea, vomiting, bradycardia, visual effects: yellow, green, or white halo around objects, decreased consciousness, abdominal pain and diarrhoea. ECG shows junctional tachycardia, PVCs, AV block, and sometimes PSVT.

14. Investigations: (P/E: Vitals, orthostatic BP, check for signs of dehydration—thirst, mucous membrane moistness, HR, urine output, skin turgor, BP; cardiopulmonary exam, neurological exam). Digoxin level, CBC, lytes, Bun, Cr, INR/PTT, glucose, ECG, 24 hr Holter monitor, echocardiogram, EEG, CT head, carotid Doppler.

Vomiting

Case 1: 40 years old man comes complaining of vomiting for 10 days.
Case 2: 55 years old known alcoholic is coming complaining of vomiting and abdominal pain for the last 12 hrs.

1.   If there is more than 1 GI complains, analyze them separately. It is easier you to get the Dx. At the end, establish the relationship between the symptoms.
2.   OCD: When did you start? How many times a day? Is it worse in the morning/evening/night?
3.   Analyze: How many cups? Undigested food from previous days? Blood? Bile-stained? Coffee ground?
4.   Character: Projectile, preceded by nausea, retching.
5.   Precipitating factors: meal, drugs, stress, certain food, alcohol.
6.   Associated symptoms: abdominal pain: (PQRST), fever, diarrhea, anorexia, heartburn, melena, weight loss, early satiety, fullness, abdominal distention, jaundice, dark urine, headaches.
7.   Analyze the sequence of occurrence: Short bowel—pain, vomiting, obstipation; Long bowel—obstipation, vomiting, pain.
8.   PMH: PUD, Crohn's, UC, abdominal surgery, DM, heart disease, kidney disease, brain tumors, anemia, pancreatic disease, gallbladder disease.
9.   Did you have any investigations because of these symptoms? Any treatment?
10. If the patient is a woman of childbearing age, always ask about pregnancy.
11. Allergies, Medications (Tums, mylant, zantac, aspirin, steroids).
12. Smoking, alcohol, drugs, travels, hepatitis, transfusions, HIV, occupations, others with the same symptoms, diet.
13. Family H/o.

Cases:
1. Gastric outlet obstruction 2. Mallory Weiss.

Jaundice

Case 1: 40 year old man comes with a week H/o of jaundice.
Case 2: 65 year old man comes with 3 weeks H/o of jaundice.
Case 3: 50 year old man known alcoholic comes complaining of jaundice.

1. OCD: When did you notice that your skin was yellow?
2. Who noticed it?
3. Did you feel well before the jaundice appears?
4. Ask the color of stools and urine
5. Pain, fever, pruritis.
6. Nausea, vomiting, anorexia, diarrhea, constipation, weight loss, increase in the abdominal girth, ankle swelling, clots in legs, joint pain, skin rash, depression.
7. Ask about risk factors/diseases causing jaundice.
8. IV drugs, blood transfusion (before 1989).
9. Alcohol, travels, exposure to hepatitis.
10. Vaccinations, occupation, diet, seafood during the last 6 weeks.
11. Smoking, unprotected sex—prostitute, homosexual, HIV patient.
12. Previous H/o of hepatitis (if yes, serology known?)
13. PMH: IBD, pancreatitis, gallstones, previous Sx, TB, hemophilia, BCP, medications: (INH, NSAIDS, diuretics, aldomet, dilantin).
14. Congenital hyperbilirubinemias (e.g. Gilbert's disease).
15. Family H/o.
16. Also think based on etiology:
    Infectious—sea food, transfusion before 1989, sexual practice (homo, prostitute)
    Obstructive—gall stones, carcinoma.
    Hemolytic—hereditary, drugs, fava beans
17. Is the cause of jaundice pre-hepatic, hepatic, post-hepatic?
18. How sick is this patient? Should s/he be admitted? Why? Explain it to the patient.
19. If there is an infectious issue, think about the patient's close contacts, returning to work and reporting the to public health authorities.
20. If ascitis/encephalopathy is positive, ask if the pants fit tighter?
21. Have you noticed an increased in the abdominal girth? Was it sudden/progressive? symmetric/asymmetric? location? sequence? swollen legs? SOB?
22. Do you have difficulty sleeping? (Alert at night/sleepy during the day? Both these are indicative of encephalopathy).
23. Bad taste in your mouth? Shaken hands?

24. Constipation, diuretics, sedatives, bleeding and infections can precipitate encephalopathy.
25. NSAIDS can cause hepato-renal syndrome.
26. Associations:
    a. Hepatic disease: Fever, jaundice, N/V, RUQ pain, melena, hematemesis, easy bruising, rash, anorexia.
    b. Encephalopathy: Insomnia, bad taste, tremor, confusion, bleeding, constipation, drugs, diet.
    c. Malignancy: Weight loss, fever, lumps, abdominal pain, anorexia, change in bowel habits.
    d. SBP: Confusion, fever, abdominal pain, rapid progression of ascitis, jaundice.
    e. CHF: Fatigue, SOB, orthopnea, nocturia, palpitations.

Cases
1. Hepatitis B
2. Pancreatic cancer.
3. Alcoholic hepatitis

Case 4: A 50 yr old man is denied life insurance because of abnormal liver function tests. AST > ALT (both elevated). AP slightly elevated, bilirubin normal. Take H/o. Give D/d. What investigations would you order?

1. H/o: Jaundice, hepatitis, foreign travel, blood transfusion, recreational IV drug use.
2. Dark urine, pale stool, abdominal pain, fever/chills, decreased appetite, weight loss.
3. Night sweats, nausea and vomiting, pruritis, easy bruising, gynecomastia, hemorrhoids (from portal hypertension), alcohol use.
4. Sexual H/o: Number of past and present partners, genders of same, STDs.
5. Medications, drug use, smoking, allergies, PMH, family H/o, ROS.
6. CAGE questionnaire:
    a. Have you tried to cut down on your alcohol?
    b. Have you ever felt angry when someone suggested you to reduce alcohol intake?
    c. Have you ever felt guilty about your drinking?
    d. Do you take an eye-opener drink in the morning?

7. DDx: Alcoholic liver disease, viral hepatitis, liver cancer—primary/metastatic.

8. Investigations: Viral serology (Hep A, B, C antibody and B antigen for > 6 months indicates chronic carrier state), GGT, AST, ALT, Alk. Phosphatase, LDH, bilirubin, INR, PTT, albumin, glucose (cirrhosis), serum ceruloplasmin, serum copper (Wilson's disease), serum ferritin, TIBC (for hemochromatosis), ANA, anti-smooth muscle antibody (autoimmune hepatitis—chronic active hepatitis), abdominal ultrasound, liver biopsy.

GI bleeding

Case 1: 46 year old man comes to ER because of malena for 10 days.
Case 2: 58 year old known alcoholic is brought by paramedics to ER because of hematemesis.
Case 3: 68 years old man comes to hospital because of bleeding per rectum for 3 days.

As soon as you start every station when somebody is bleeding, assume that the patient is unstable hemodynamically, so assess your ABCs and volume status and make sure that the patient is stable before starting your interview.

1. OCD: Ask directly to the patient: How do you feel?
2. Dizzy? Did you pass out? Palpitations?
3. When did it start? Sudden onset?
4. Color—Bright red/coffee grounds/black?
5. Consistency, amount in cups, every stool?
6. Bad smell? Stool caliber?
7. Diarrhea/constipation?
8. Associated symptoms: When bleeding develops rapidly, body gets very less time to compensate and therefore most symptomatic. Chronic conditions may present insidiously.
9. Anemia/hypovolemia: dizziness, light headedness, palpitations, fatigue, hematemesis, hematuria, hematochezia.
10. Malignancy: Abdominal pain (PQRST), weight loss, ascitis, anorexia, dysphagia, lumps.
11. PUD: Heartburn, dyspepsia, N/V, H/o of NSAIDs, PMH of PUD.
12. Alcohol related bleeding: retching-vomiting before, previous OGDs, H/o of varices, bleeding, stigmata of alcoholic liver disease.
13. PMH: PUD, bleeding disorders, liver disease, kidney diseases, DM, HTN, heart problems.
14. Medications: NSAIDS, blood thinners, steroids, iron.
15. Allergies group and type if known.
16. Previous transfusions.
17. Alcohol, smoking, drugs, occupation, diet, travels, country of immigration.
18. Family H/o: Cancer, bleeding tendencies, PUD, liver disorders.
19. Conclude the interview explaining that he has to be admitted.
20. Start with upper OGD and then if normal do lower endoscopy.

Management
1. ABCs
2. O$_2$/IV fluids/monitor
3. O$_2$ saturation
4. Vitals every 5min, assess orthostatic changes
5. Cardiac monitor Intravenous access (2 short large bore 14 gauge in antecubital area).
6. Start with fluid resuscitation crystalloids/ringer lactate bolus and assess permanently (expect to need approximately 3 times the estimated blood loss—rule of 3:1).
7. Cross and type 6 units of packed RBCs as soon as possible. Start if non-responsive after 2-3 L of fluids. In severe s start with non-cross matched O negative packed RBCs. Fresh Frozen Plasma (FFP) if coagulation defects.
8. If active control of hemorrhage is needed, do not wait until the patient is stable, call surgery and or GI.
9. Now that the patient out of shock, ask for the work up: CBC, INR, PT, PTT, lytes, Ca, Mg, PO$_4$, albumin, RFT, LFT, ECG, X-ray, ABGs.
10. Drugs: Pantolac 80 mg bolus, then 8 mg/h, IV vasopressin.
11. When the patient is stable, OGD, balloon, other procedures.
12. Constant assessment is the clue in management.
13. If hemorrhagic shock, direct your treatment accordingly.
14. Foley's catheter and input/output chart.

Cases:
1. PUD 2. Esophageal varices 3. Diverticulitis.

Diarrhea

Case 1: 0 year old woman with diarrhea 3 weeks.
Case 2: 26 year old woman with bloody diarrhea 10 days.
Case 3: 28 year old man HIV positive comes with diarrhea 1 month.
Case 4: 48 year old known alcoholic complains of diarrhea and weight loss.

1. OCD: Make sure that this is diarrhea
2. How long have you before having diarrhea?
3. How many bowel movements a day? Sudden onset? Intermittent?
4. Loose stools/constipation?
5. Is it getting worse? New symptoms?
6. Not able to keep anything down?
7. How many times do you have to go to the washroom?
8. Color: Bloody? mucus, pus, greenish, pale
9. Amount: watery, med, bulky, greasy (hard to flush the toilet?)
10. Odor: foul.
11. Timing: morning, the whole day, do you wake up during the night?
12. Aggravating/relieving factors: meals, certain foods (dairy products, vegetables) stress, drugs (laxatives).
13. Abdominal pain (PQRST), fever, chills, N/V, anorexia, weight loss, flatulance-belching-passing gas.
14. Tenesumus.
15. Do you feel the urge to go to the washroom and to strain with little result?
16. Do you have to rash to go to the toilet and some time you can not make it—incontinence)
17. Can you keep anything in your stomach or just go through?
18. Joint pain, rash, vision changes, night blindness, kidney/gallbladder stones, mouth ulcers, easy bruising, lumps, heat intolerance, palpitations, neck swelling.
19. Source of infection: Did you eat outside?
20. Sea food, home made food?
21. Others sick too? Travel any where? (Establish timing in between returning and the developing of symptoms)
22. Medication: Antibiotics during the last 6 weeks, allergies.
23. PMH: liver, IBD, PUD, hyperthyroidism, DM, previous infections, carrier if coming from different countries.
24. Alcohol, smoking, drugs, HIV, occupation:
25. How is this problem affecting your every day activities?
26. Are you able to continue working? Did you have to take day off?

This can be a vague station, but also think that the patient can be anxious and very sick. So evaluate how serious the condition is and go to the following points:

1. Is this an acute process or a chronic one (> 4 weeks)?
2. Do you think that the patient needs hospitalization-the patient looks dehydrated, toxic, malnourished, lost weight?
3. If you need to order tests, haw fast do you need them, explain to the patient what to do in the mean time.
4. Can the patient go back to work, if you suspect an infectious and contagious disease?
5. Explain if any treatment (diet, antibiotics, anti-diarrhoeal medications).
6. Think if you need to assess the patient's close contacts to R/o infection.
7. Think if you need to report to Public Heath.

Cases:
1: Pseudo-membranous colitis
2: IBD (probably UC)
3: HIV associated diarrhea: MAC, Cryptosporidium, CMV.
4: Malabsorption

Case 5: 19 yr old female with chronic diarrhoea. Take H/o.

1. Crohn's, ulcerative colitis, irritable bowel syndrome, malabsorption (celiac disease, tropical sprue), lactose intolerance, intestinal infection (C.difficile, Giardia, Amoebiasis), pancreatic dysfunction, unusual diet, laxative abuse.
2. H/o: Onset of diarrhoea, duration, consistency and colour of stools, do they float?
3. Is there blood or mucous? Frequency of BMs/day, weight loss, appetite.
4. Dietary H/o: Is diarrhoea worse with milk? (Lactose intolerance tends to produce explosive diarrhoea after milk ingestion—hereditary), laxative use.
5. Use of antibiotics in the past 6 weeks.
6. Travel H/o. Fever, nausea, vomiting, infectious illnesses.
7. Associated abdominal pain, fatigue, uveitis, mouth or anal ulcers.
8. Ankylosing spondylitis, sacroilitis, renal problems (due to malabsorption), arthritis (these are associated with Crohn's).
9. Malnutrition signs/symptoms: lassitude, weakness, hair falling out, skin rash, easy bruising, weight loss, anaemia.
10. Neurological findings (confusion, emotional lability, loss of vibration and position sense), glossitis.

11. Medications, drugs, alcohol, smoking (decreases risk and symptoms of inflammatory bowel disease).
12. PMH (IBD, abdominal surgery), family H/o, ROS.

Case 6: 21 year old female with bloody diarrhoea. Take H/o.

1. Abdominal cramping. 6 watery stools during the past 4 hrs.
2. Contain maroon-coloured blood. Feels dizzy and weak.
3. No previous H/o of diarrhoea, previously well.
4. OCD. Frequency.
5. Appearance of stools: How well formed, is bright red or dark brown-black blood on or mixed with stools.
6. Pain with bowel movements, abdominal pain or cramps with location, radiation, precipitating factors and alleviating factors, quality, severity, timing with respect to defecation, gas, bloating, heart burn, peptic ulcer, reflux, hiatus hernia.
7. Extra-intestinal features of IBD: Iritis, arthritis, mouth ulcers, anal ulcers, skin lesions, kidney stones.
8. Infectious diarrhoea: Inquire about fever, nausea, vomiting, weight loss, fatigue, recent travel, consumption of unusual foods or foods which may have been contaminated.
9. Recent intake of antibiotics.
10. Family members sick at home, pelvic pain, vaginal bleeding, and vaginal discharge.
11. Past medical H/o, medications (e.g. NSAIDS), family H/o of IBDs, familial polyposis, review of systems.
12. Investigations: CBC with differential, stool for ova, parasites and culture, C. Difficile toxin, endoscopy (from above first).
13. Type and cross match for 4 units of PRBCs.
14. D/d: 1. Gastroenteritis, 2. Bleeding peptic ulcer, 3. Inflammatory bowel disease.

Stroke

Case1: 68 years old man is brought to ER because of sudden onset of right side weakness.
Case2: 70 years old woman comes to ER because of 2 episodes of sudden weakness at the right side of her body that resolved spontaneously in 5 min. today.
Case3: 65 years old woman presents in ER because of sudden onset of dysarthria and right hand weakness.

Make sure that the patient is stable. Check ABC.

O—When did you notice the weakness? Sudden/gradually installed? What were you doing?

C—Are the symptoms getting worse? From paresis to plegia? LOC?

D—Duration (thrombolysis may be offered in the first 3 hrs)

1. Weakness: In face, arm, and leg.
2. Speech: Dysarthria v/s aphasias
3. Sensory symptoms: Anesthesia, hypoesthesia, paresthesias. Gait problems:
4. Associated symptoms:
   a. Anterior cerebral artery—clumsiness, aphasia, incontinence
   b. Middle cerebral artery—homonymous hemianopia, sensory defects
   c. Posterior cerebral artery—loss of vision (one or both homonymous visual fields)
   d. Vertebral artery—ataxia, vertigo, diplopia, dysphagia, dysarthria.

5. Risk factors: HTN, DM, smoking, hypercholesterolemia, AF, valvular diseases.
6. PMH: Previous strokes, RF, peripheral vascular diseases, hematological diseases, cancer.
7. Medications: Anti-HTN, anticoagulation, aspirin, cardiac meds.
8. Social: Smoking, alcohol, drugs, occupation, diet, hobbies, family support, ADL/IADL.
9. Family H/o: Stroke, MI, sudden death.
10. Determine if the patient can be included in the protocol for thrombolysis.
11. Evolution: TIA, stroke in evolution, completed stroke.

If you have to examine the patient:
1. ABCs and ask vitals
2. Orientation to place, person and time
3. Inspection: Position, posture, asymmetries, gaze deviations, dysarthria/slurred speech/aphasia.
4. CNS—Cranial nerves:

II—PEARL, gross visual acuity, screening confrontation, accommodation, swing light test, fundoscopy.

III, IV, VI—Occular movements, ptosis, nistagmus, diplopia, eye deviation

V—Clench your teeth (temporal), sensation

VI—Corneal reflex

VII—Wrinkle your head, keep your eyes close, blow your checks, smile.

VIII—Hearing: whisper a number, can you repeat it (distract at the same time). Rinne/Weber.

IX—Open your mouth: say ah-ah, Gag reflex

X—Soft palate-position, uvula.

XI—Shrug your shoulders; push your head against my hands to the sides.

XII—Stick out your tongue

5. Motor: Tone, power (muscle groups)
6. Reflexes: All common ones and also include primitive reflexes
7. Sensation: sharp/dull; light touch, vibration, position, discrimination (stereognosis, graphiestesia, 2 point discrimination, 2 point localization, extinction).
8. Cerebellar exam.
9. CVS exam (AF, murmurs, carotid bruits)
10. Brain stem reflexes: Doll's eye, caloric tests.

Cases: 1. MCA stroke. 2. Crescendo TIA. 3. ACA stroke

Movement disorders

Case1: 60 years old woman comes to your office complaining of tremor of the left arm. Examine
Case2: 34 years old man known schizophrenic in long term treatment with neuroleptic develops abnormal movements. Examine the patient.

1. Introduction: Explain to the patient what you are going to do.
2. Ask the vitals (orthostatic dropping).
3. Inspection: Look for abnormal postures, distress, sitting, lying.
4. Face: blinking, oculogyric crisis, convergence decrease, mouth lip smacking, tongue movements, tics, facial grimacing, head titubation, torticolis, dystonias.
5. Hands: Tremor (pill-rolling, fine, coarse, at rest, intentional), chorea, athetosis, hemibalism, myoclonias—Legs: akathisia. Gait: Stand wide based? Neck flexion.
6. Gait: Type (festinant, scissors, spastic), tendency to fall.
7. Parkinson: Shuffling steps, increase in speed, trouble initiating and turning. Cerebellar: tandem, unstable, falls towards the affected side. Speech: monotonus, dysarthria, say "British constitution", slurred, scanty, explosive (cerebellar).
8. Writing test: Ask the patient to draw a spiral shape. Cerebellar (large spiral); Parkinson (small spiral).
9. Tone: Cogwheel (Parkinson); Lead pipe rigidity (Parkinson); Hypotonia (cerebellar)
10. Reflexes—Pendular in cerebellar
11. Coordination: Dysmetry, rapid alternating movements (dyadiadocokinesia), heal to shin-Cerebellar
12. Drift-Lateral and downward-cerebellar
13. Nistagmus
14. Motor strength.
15. Cerbellar features: Fall to one side, draws large spiral, tells "British Constitution" with an explosive voice, hypotonia, pendular reflexes.

Cases:
1: Parkinson disease 2: Dystonia related to neuroleptics

Case3: 64 yr old woman with resting tremor. Perform focussed P/E.

1. Parkinson's disease: Resting tremor, rigidity, akinesia/bradykinesia, postural instability, mask-like face.

2. Vitals.
3. Observe patient at rest: Pill-rolling tremor in the upper limb which is worst at rest, may also have head tremor (titubation), stooped posture, open-mouthed, mask-like face, generally hypokinetic with decreased blinking and noticeable drooling.
4. MMSE: Dementia associated with Parkinson's (50% of patients), may find poor short-term memory, poor concentration, abstraction, micrographia.
5. Depression may also present.
6. Cranial nerves, body power, pronator drift, deep tendon reflexes and Babinski are normal in Parkinson's.
7. Tone: Bilateral lead pipe (constant), rigidity with possible cog-wheeling due to tremor superimposed on passive motion. Test elbow, forearm rotation and knee by applying rapid passive motion while feeling the muscle tendon.
8. Cerebellar testing: Finger-nose and heel-shin tests show improvement of tremor with intention (i.e. resting tremor rather than an intention tremor), rapid alternating movements are poor bilaterally in Parkinson's and Rhomberg's is positive due to postural instability.
9. The Parkinsonian gait is unsteady and shuffling with small steps, decreased arm swinging, and a tendency to fall forward or backward.
10. Tries to increase forward speed to keep from falling (festinant gait).

Hoarseness

Case1: 60 year old man comes to your office complaining of a 2-month H/o of hoarseness. Take focused H/o.
Case2: 45 year old woman comes to the clinic complaining of hoarseness. Take H/o.

1. Clarify what does the patient mean by hoarseness?
2. Onset of symptoms: When did you notice that your voice change?
3. Is it bi-tonal voice? Can the patient talk? Dysphonia?
4. Did any one tell you that you sound hoarse? Did you realize?
5. Is it getting worse? Is it present all the time? Morning? Is it related to stress?
6. Medications? Is it progressive? Is it fluctuating?
7. Duration: Did it present out of the blue (stroke)? Progressive? Since when?
8. Infections: Fever, sore throat, cough, lymphadenopathies
9. Cancer: Hoarseness and then dysphagia: Larynx cancer
10. Dysphagia and then hoarseness: Esophageal cancer, weight loss, dysphonia, decrease in appetite, hemoptysis, foreign body sensation, lumps in the neck.
11. GER: Heartburn, ear pain, sore throat, wheezing, sore sensation in the mouth, vomiting.
12. Hypothyroidism: neck swelling, tiredness, constipation, skin dryness, depression, weight gain.
13. PMH: Lung diseases, PUD, thyroid conditions, liver disease, traumas, TB infection, intubations, ENT problems, immuno-suppressive conditions? (chemotherapy, HIV, cancer)
14. Medications, allergies.
15. Occupation/hobbies: Do you use your voice to work? Sing?
16. Social H/o: Smoking, alcohol, drugs, contact with irritants, anybody sick around you?
17. Work description; how much is this problem affecting the patient's every day's life?
18. Risk factors for HIV?
19. Family H/o: Lung-larynx cancer, other conditions related.
20. Key points: Stroke, oesphageal reflux, ear pain, intubations, chemotherapy, cancer, singer, lye ingestion, smoking, dysphagia, dysphonia, dyspnoea.

Alzheimer's disease

Case1: Mrs. X is a 45 year old woman who came to talk to you about her mother. She says that her mother has not been herself lately. Interview her.

Case2: Mr. X is a 68 year old man who came today to talk to you because he feels fatigued. He is now taking care of his wife at home. Interview him.

Case3: Mr. X is a 62 year old man who comes to your office for the results of neuropsychological and neurological testing. According to the neurologist, Mr. X has a clinical presentation of Alzheimer's disease. Interview him and address his questions.

1. Start your interview with an open question. What is the main concern? Why did the patient decide to come today? If the patient is not present, ask why the patient is not present?
2. Start taking your H/o: Do not mention the name "Alzheimer". Ask if you are the first one to be consulted? Ask how close the daughter is with the mother; are they living together? Is she in a nursing home, retirement home?
3. Start with the cognitive assessment: I am going to ask you a few questions regarding your mother, wife. Start with ADL/IADL that gives you an idea of recent changes in the patient's level of functioning. Establish the changes in function over the time (last year/6 ms). Is this progressive/gradual, step wise, sudden?
4. Continue with warning signs. Memory: have you noticed that your mother/wife has difficulties remembering things? Is more forgetful, especially with things that happen more recently? Learning new information? Forgetting recent events, loosing the keys, phone #, names, (old memory is preserved).
5. Difficulties performing familiar tasks: Unable to prepare meals that were used to do? Gets recipes, ingredients.
6. Problems with language: Trouble finding the right word?
7. Disorientation in time and place: Become lost in their own street?
8. Decreased judgment: Dressing inappropriately for the weather, inappropriate comments.
9. Problems with abstract thinking: Ask "What is a birthday party?"
10. Misplacing things: Sweater in the freezer, watch in the sugar bowl.
11. Changes in mood or behavior: Mood swings without reason.
12. Changes in personality: Confusion, withdrawn, agitated, suspicious.
13. Delusions/hallucinations.
14. Loss of initiative: Passive but active before.
15. PMH: To R/U secondary causes of dementia.
16. Vascular D: Stroke, HTN, step wise decline.

17. Parkinson's: Tremor, rigidity, akinesia, postural hypotension.
18. Anemia (B12): Low Hb, neurological symptoms, fatigue, gastric problems,
19. Hypothyroidism: Weight gain, cold intolerance, changes in voice, dry skin.
20. Infections: Previous H/o of syphilis, encephalitis.
21. HIV: Risk factors, opportunistic infections.
22. Hydrocephalus: Ataxia, incontinence, dementia.
23. Alcohol related dementia: H/o of alcohol intake, Wernicke-Korsakoff.
24. Pseudodementia: H/o of depression.
25. Trauma associated injuries: Head injuries in the past.
26. Other systemic diseases: DM, CTD, renal/hepatic failure, brain tumors, CHF, sarcoidosis.
27. Medications, allergies, alcohol, drugs, social H/o, and occupation.
28. Brief psychiatry screen (1/6 of Alzheimer's patients have depression, 1/3 present psychosis).
29. Family H/o: Dementia, psychiatric diseases.
30. Open questions to the patient, expectations, ideas of what seems to be wrong.
31. Key points: ADLs, IADLs, learning new information, retrograde amnesia for recent stuff, mood, delusion (1/3), drugs. Don't use the word "Alzheimer" for 6 months.

1. Explain that you need to see the patient to do a full P/E and MMSE
2. Do not talk about Alzheimer yet, although some features point the disease, you need time (at least 6 months) and test (to R/o) other conditions before.
3. If the patient asks you in particular about Alzheimer's, give a brief explanation of the condition. Explain that there will be chronic deterioration.
4. Offer support, groups, information, F/U.

Dealing with difficult situations

Case1: Ms. X is a 30 year old man who came to talk to you regarding his Crohn's disease. You are going to meet him for the first time. Interview.

Case2: Mr. Y is a 45 year old man immigrant from Bosnia who is coming to see you because he cannot sleep and feels irritable. Talk to him.

Case3: Mr. Z is a 37 year old man who comes to see you to talk about his wife. She is your patient, but he is not. She has left the house and he is looking for her. Talk to him.

Case4: Mrs. A is a 40 year old woman whose father has just passed away this morning during a complicated AAA surgery. She is "very angry" saying that she did not expect this to happen. Talk to her.

1. Be ready the patient to jump when you less expected
2. Start taking your H/o till the patient becomes very angry or start screaming or swearing. Keep it cool, do not intervene, and let him/her open up the problem.
3. When the times comes, start gently addressing that you see how frustrated the patient is Use de-escalating techniques: keeping normal/calming tone of voice even if the patient screams. Sooner or later the patient is going to come down.
4. Try to find out why the patient is angry, after all, there is always a reason to be angry.
5. Explore the problem deeply. Find out how much this distress the patient's life.
6. Explore the family situation, workplace, finances, relationships, addictions.
7. Offer help, counseling, talk to the family group.
8. Remember, the fact that you are trying to help. It does not mean that you have to agree in everything the patient wants. Be gentle but firm in your position.

Cases:
1. Wife's gambling
2. Depression secondary to family situation (wife with terminal colon cancer)
3. Woman that ran away because of abuse.
4. Anger because of unexpected death of a loved one

Needle prick

Case: OR nurse sustained needle stick injury. Worried about hepatitis and AIDS. Counsel.

1. Determine the severity of exposure: Hollow ore needle?
2. Needle gauge? Depth of penetration? Did needle contain blood from a patient?
3. Was any blood injected? Is the HIV and hepatitis status of the patient known?
4. Is the nurse immunized for hepatitis B?
5. Odds of transmission HIV (0.3%); Hep B Antigen (40%); Hep C Antibody (10%).
6. Hep. B causes fulminant hepatic necrosis in 1% of those infected, which is fatal in 60%.
7. 5% of those infected with Hep.B remain in a chronic carrier state, which is associated with a 25-40% risk of cirrhosis and hepatocellular cancer.
8. There is a 50% risk of chronic liver disease once infected with Hep C. The risks of cirrhosis and hepatocellular cancer are similar to those for Hep B.
9. Recommend baseline testing for HIV, Hep B and C in nurse and patient (require consent for HIV testing).
10. If the patient was recently infected, he may not become positive on antigenic testing for up to 3 months. Therefore, nurse and patient should be retested.
11. Recommend HIV prophylaxis (AZT + 3TC x 4 weeks) for significant needle stick from a patient with known HIV or who is a high risk (multiple partners, IV drug user, anal intercourse, recent immigrant from endemic area).
12. If the nurse is not effectively immunized (i.e. antibody titres tested) against Hep B, recommend immunization.
13. If patient is found to be Hep B or C positive, give the nurse passive immunity gamma globulin.
14. Hep B gamma globulin within seven days of exposure has been proven to be effective in preventing transmission.

Hypertension

Case: 20 yr old female with hypertension. Perform a P/E. Give a DDx. What investigations would you order?

1. 4 limb BP for coarctation of the aorta (look for delayed pulse and decreased BP in legs, also harsh systolic murmur radiating to the back).
2. Examine fundi for hypertensive damage.
3. Renal bruits for renal artery stenosis.
4. Signs of hyperthyroidism: Lid retraction, lid lag, globe lag, exophthalmos, goitre, tachycardia, widened pulse pressure, skin is warm, fine, moist, fine tremor, nervousness, hyperactivity, DTR.
5. Cushing's disease: Moon facies, buffalo hump, striae, mood disorder.
6. DDx:
    a. Idiopathic (still the most common), renal artery stenosis due to fibromuscular hyperplasia or atherosclerosis.
    b. Renal parenchymal disease: Drugs (NSAIDs, OCP, gentamycin), glomerulonephritis.
    c. Endocrine: Hyperthyroidism, pheochromocytoma, hyperaldosteronism due to adrenal hyperfunction, Cushing's, Coarctation of aorta.
7. Initial Investigations: Lytes, BUN, Cr, TSH.

Case: 23 yr old with BP 160/100 in both arms. Perform a focussed P/E. Give four possible diagnoses. What four investigations would you order? If these investigations were negative, give two steps in your initial management plan.

1. Patient should be disrobed to underwear, and draped below the waist.
2. P/E for hypertension: Combines exams for atherosclerosis, coarctation, hyperthyroidism, and Cushing's disease.
3. Patient Sitting: Take vitals (need BP in all 4 limbs—do legs when lying down). Inspect for cyanosis, arcus senilis in the eyes (sign of high cholesterol), bulging veins in the upper chest (SVC syndrome), supraclavicular fat pad, buffalo hump, moon face, truncal obesity, striae, nicotine stains on fingers, clubbing, flame hemorrhages on nails, obesity, high work of breathing, intercostal indrawing, symmetric chest movement, visible apex beat.
4. Fundoscopy for retinopathy of hypertension: (in order of increasing severity of
    damage)—constriction and sclerosis of retinal arterioles, hemorrhages, exudates,
    papilloedema.

5. Thyroid exam: Inspect patient for proptosis, "thyroid state" (upper lids do not overlap the irises). Have patient follow your finger up and down to check for lid lag and globe lag. Is skin thin, dry, and flaky or diaphoretic?

6. Palpate thyroid standing behind the patient and ask them to swallow.

7. Inspect nails for leukonychia and hands for tremor (can place a piece of paper on the hand held horizontal to detect fine tremor).

8. Check biceps reflexes with thumb held over tendon; feel for slow phase reflex of hypothyroidism. Hyperthyroid nails: "Plummer's nails"—soft with onycholysis.

9. Palpate the apex, note whether it is laterally displaced (lateral to the mid-clavicular line) and feel for thrill or heave, feel radial pulses in the arms simultaneously, note any delay.

10. Percuss the lung fields anteriorly and posteriorly.

11. Auscultate the lung fields anteriorly and posteriorly, listen to the heart in the mitral (apex, 5th interspace, mid-clavicular line), tricuspid (right sternal border, 5th interspace), pulmonic (left sternal border, 2nd interspace) and aortic (right sternal border, 2nd interspace) areas as well as over the right clavicle, and both carotids. Listen for rub. To bring out an aortic murmur (typically aortic regurgitation) and coarctation bruits, ask patient to lean forward, exhale and stop breathing while you listen over the aortic and pulmonic areas.

12. Patient lying: Auscultate for bruits over the renal arteries. Observe for pulsations due to AAA, palpate abdomen for hepatomegaly. Palpate femoral pulses, and auscultate for femoral bruits, palpate the popliteal pulses, inspect the legs and feet for venous stasis or arterial insufficiency ulcers, palpate the dorsalis pedis and tibialis posterior pedal pulses. Feel the ankle for pitting edema.

13. Tibial BP: BP cuff placed around calf, auscultate the tibialis posterior pulse posterior to the medial malleolus.

14. JVP: Raise the head of the bed 30 degrees and inspect the neck. A jugular venous pulsation higher than 4 cm ASA is abnormal.

15. Check the hepato-jugular reflux (compress the liver, the JVP should either not rise or remain elevated only transiently).

16. D/d: Essential hypertension, renal artery insufficiency, drug-induced (thyroid hormone and OCP) and coarctation of the aorta.

Rx for hypertension:
1. Target 140/90; if DM or Renal: <125/75
2. Rx until 2 readings are less than target.

3. Lifestyle changes-smoking-alcohol-wt if BMI >25/aerobic excercise 30 min 4 times a week.
4. Cognitive intervention if stressed.
5. Diet.
6. Pharmacology—If dBP>90 with target organ damage—first line monotherapy with any one of the 4 (thiazide (monitor K), beta blocker, ACE inhibitor, Ca channel blocker).
7. If no use combination of CCB + ACEI or beta blocker/Diuretic + ACE or beta blocker.
8. Isolated systolic hypertension—thiazide low dose or CCB.
9. IHD—beta blocker, ACE inhibitor
10. DM—ACE inhibitor
11. Asthma—K sparing + thiazide diuretics for patients on salbutamol
12. Pregnancy—Methyl DOPA
13. Hypertensive emergency—Labetalol or nifidipine

Fatigue

Case: 40 yr old female with fatigue. Take H/o. Findings: cold intolerance, weight gain.

1. Fatigue H/o: Onset, chronology, past episodes, functional limitations, associated with exertion?
2. Recent viral illness (mononucleosis), cold intolerance, weight gain, dry skin, brittle hair, hoarseness (hypothyroidism), associated muscle aches (fibromyalgia), chest pain (angina), SOB (CHF), sleep and depression H/o.
3. Medications (TCAs, sedatives, antihypertensives), drug/alcohol use, allergies, smoking, PMH, family H/o, ROS.
4. Diagnosis: Most likely hypothyroidism given cold intolerance and weight gain.
5. Etiology: Pneumonics: PS VINDICATE
    Psychogenic: Depression/sleep disorders/life stresses/anxiety/chronic fatigue syndrome
    Sedentary
    Vascular: Stroke
    Infectious: Viral (infectious mononucleosis, hepatitis), bacterial (TB), fungal, parasitic
    HIV
    Neoplastic
    Nutrition: Anemia, B12 deficiency
    Neurogenic: Myesthenia, MS
    Drugs: Beta blockers, antihistamine, anticholinergics, diazepam, antiepileptics
    Idiopathic
    Chronic Illness: CHF, COPD, RF
    Autoimmune: SLE, RA, and MCTD
    Toxin: Substance abuse, alcohol, heavy metal poisoning
    Endocrine: Hypothyroidism, DM, Cushing's, adrenal insufficiency, pregnancy

Impotence

Case: 47 yr old male with impotence. Wants "pills" for this. Fears losing girlfriend. Take H/o and counsel.

1. The causes of erectile dysfunction are subdivided into functional and organic categories in a 1:1 ratio.
2. The problem is rarely primary (i.e. "never had ability to sustain erection").
3. Impotence is defined as the inability to have satisfactory intercourse due to erectile dysfunction in at least 25% of encounters.
4. The organic causes are:
   a. Drugs—(beta blockers, thiazides, H2-blockers, antidepressants, antipsychotics, digoxin, clofibrate, sedatives, alcohol, heroin)
   b. Hormones (prolactin-secreting pituitary tumour, associated with loss of libido and testicular atrophy), neurogenic (stroke, DM, MS, surgery, radiation, spinal cord injury)
   c. Vascular (peripheral vascular disease, DM, hypertension, surgery or radiation)
5. H/o: Current partners. Problems in relationships.
6. Why is the patient seeking medical attention for this now?
7. H/o—Onset of erectile dysfunction and chronology.
8. Description of the problem: No erection at all, cannot sustain erection, ejaculate too quickly to satisfy partner, cannot achieve orgasm or orgasm without ejaculation, retrograde ejaculation.
9. Circumstances under which impotence occurs: only with certain partners, only at certain times or locations, what percentage of the time?
10. Is impotence related to lack of sexual desire?
11. Presence and firmness of morning or nocturnal erections.
12. Does the patient sustain erections during masturbation?
13. Associated problems: Anxiety attacks, anhedonia, perineal or peripheral numbness, poor peripheral circulation.
14. Exercise, medications, contraceptive method, drug use, smoking, cholesterol, allergies, PMH, past surgical H/o, family H/o, ROS.
15. Counselling: Discuss causes of impotence in terms of organic v/s inorganic aetiology, and that it tends to cause great anxiety, normalize patient's feelings.
16. Erectile dysfunction can often be improved with lifestyle changes: exercise, weight loss, improved diet, decreased alcohol intake, smoking cessation, stress management, sleep hygiene, better diabetes control, joint counselling with partner to decrease anxiety. Improvement of patient's relationship with partner: address sexual boredom.

17. Review medications: Suggest changes.
18. Explain that many organic causes of impotence are unfortunately not reversible.
19. Describe therapeutic options.
20. Counselling with partner or alternative means of sexual gratification.
21. Testosterone preparations or bromocryptine (for prolactinoma) if patient is shown to have hormonal disturbance on blood work (measure testosterone and gonadotropins).
22. Viagra, vacuum-rubber ring device, penile prostheses.
23. Arrange follow-up with both partners.

Cardiology P/E

Case: Middle-aged woman with systolic ejection murmur radiating into carotids. Perform P/E.

1. The P/E for a patient with a heart murmur is a cardiopulmonary exam:
2. Patient sitting: Take vitals.
3. Inspect for cyanosis, arcus senilis in the eyes (sign of high cholesterol), bulging veins in the upper chest (SVC syndrome), nicotine stains on fingers, clubbing, flame hemorrhages on nails, obesity, work of breathing, intercostal indrawing, symmetric chest movement, visible apex beat.
4. Palpate the apex, note whether it if laterally displaced (lateral to the mid-clavicular line) and feet for thrill or heave, feel radial pulses bilaterally.
5. Percuss the lung fields anteriorly and posteriorly.
6. Auscultate the lung fields anteriorly and posteriorly, listen to the heart in the mitral (apex, 5th interspace, mid-clavicular line), tricuspid (right sternal border, 5th interspace), pulmonic (left sternal border, 2nd interspace) and aortic (right sternal border, 2nd interspace) areas as well as over the right clavicle, and both carotids. Listen for rub. To bring out an aortic murmur (typically aortic regurgitation, ask patient to lean forward, exhale and stop breathing while you listen over the aortic area. To bring out a mitral murmur, ask patient to lie supine and roll partly onto the left side while you listen over the apex. In general, murmurs are accentuated by increasing the dynamicity of the heart with mild exercise, such as asking the patient to lie down and get up again.
7. Innocent murmurs are <3/6 in intensity, peak early in systole, stop long before S2, are heard best at the base of the heart (aortic and pulmonic areas), are not associated with clicks or heaves, and ECG and CXR are normal.
8. Patient lying supine: Auscultate for bruits over the renal arteries in the abdomen.
9. Observe for pulsations due to AAA, palpate abdomen, femoral pulses, and auscultate for femoral bruits, palpate the popliteal pulses, inspect the legs and feet for venous stasis or arterial insufficiency ulcers, palpate the dorsalis pedis and tibialis posterior pedal pulses.
10. JVP: Raise the head of the bed 30 degrees and inspect the neck. A jugular venous pulsation higher than 4 cm ASA is abnormal and a sign of CHF or fluid overload.
11. Check the hepatojugular reflux (compress the liver, the JVP should either not rise or remain elevated only transiently).

Case: 50 yr old man with left-sided chest pain. Manage (means H/o, physical, investigations and treatment). Findings: bruises on chest wall, normal chest x-ray, and ECG.

1. H/o for chest pain: Describe the pain, location, radiation, quality, time of onset, duration, intensity, circumstances under which it occurs, aggravating and relieving factors, associated symptoms such as nausea, SOB, dizziness, diaphoresis, dependent edema, leg pain.
2. Respiratory symptoms: Cough sputum, fever, and hemoptysis.
3. GI symptoms, heartburn, dysphagia, previous episodes, and chronology of these.
4. H/o of trauma, asthma, bronchitis, COPD, pneumothorax, recent viral illness and previous chicken pox (herpes zoster can cause chest pain), gastritis, peptic ulcer, reflux.
5. Risk factors for heart and lung disease: Smoking, hypertension, hyperlipidemia.
6. PMH especially diabetes, heart disease including pericarditis, lung disease, GI problems, surgical H/o, and family H/o.
7. Medications, drug use, smoking, allergies, ROS.
8. P/E: Cardiopulmonary exam with the addition of inspection and palpation of the chest wall for traumatic or MSK pain source.
9. Investigations: CXR, ECG.
10. Treatment: Given a normal CXR and ECG with a chest wall bruise as evidence of trauma, send patient home, recommend non-prescription pain medication and advise that the pain should subside gradually.
11. Since the patient is at risk because of his age group and male gender, explain the symptoms of MI and advise to return immediately if these occur.

Portal Hypertension

Case: 25 yr old male with H/o of dyspepsia and binge drinking has abdominal pain. Perform a focussed P/E. What radiological investigations would you order and why?

1. P/E for abdominal pain: vitals, posture (unmoving in fetal position suggests peritonitis while writhing suggests renal colic), jaundice, nutritional status, buccal mucosa, teeth, breath (hepatic fetor), parotid hypertrophy, glossitis.
2. Inspect chest for telangectasia, gynecomastia, and loss of axillary hair. Hands: erythema, clubbing, Dupuytren's contracture, wasting of hand intrinsics.
3. Abdominal exam (supine): Inspect for caput medusa, pulsations, auscultate for bowel sounds, renal bruits.
4. Estimate size of liver and spleen by percussion. Palpate for liver edge, Murphy's sign (press on patient's liver edge after patient has exhaled, patient catches breath on inspiration), splenic enlargement (begin palpation of RLQ to catch very large spleen), hard stool in bowel. Note rigidity, rebound, guarding, tenderness, pain at McBurney's point (1/3 way along the line between the right anterior iliac crest and the umbilicus).
5. Rovsing's sign: palpation of the LLQ produces RLQ pain. Psoas sign: pain on passive or active flexion at the hip, indicates peritoneal irritation over the psoas or psoas abscess.
6. Obturator sign: pain on internal or external rotation of the hip, indicates bowel herniation into the obturator canal.
7. Ask patient to roll onto side and pound costovertebral angles lightly with fist. CP angle tenderness indicates kidney pain due to pyelonephritis or nephrolithiasis.
8. Palpate groins for hernias.
9. Rectal: Palpate prostate, rectal shelf, check for gross or occult blood.
10. Radiological investigations: Abdominal 3 views: Supine, upright, decubitus.
11. Dilated bowel with multiple air/fluid levels indicates ilieus. Dilated proximal bowel with collapsed distal bowel indicates obstruction.
12. Small bowel has circular plica: lines go all the way across. Large bowel has interrupted haustra: lines go halfway across
13. Check for calcified kidney stone, fecolith and appendiceal air/fluid level.
14. Look for gallstones and abdominal aortic aneurysm if calcified.
15. Abdominal U/S: Gallstones, cholecystitis, pancreatitis, appendicitis, hydronephropathy, kidney stones, abdominal aneurysm.
16. CXR: Check for free air under the diaphragm in an upright film.

Diabetes Counsel:

1. Type 1 from destruction of pancreas. Type 1 peak at 13 years
2. Type 2 from insulin resistance. Type 2 peak at 53 years. Fasting BS >7 mmol/L-HbA1C>7%.
3. Goals-To avoid complications-DKA-hyperglycemia-infection-CVA-CVD-PVD/Fasting BG-4-7mmol/L-HbA1c<7%-BP<130/80/LDL<2.5-TG<1.5-TC/HDL ratio-<4.
4. KA cause fruity smell-anorexia-N.V-fatigue-abdo. pain-Kussmaul breathing.
5. Physical-ht-wt-BMI-BP/fundoscopy—oral-thyroid/CHF-pulse/abdo.exam/hand foot skin/neurological exam.
6. Investigations: FBS-HbA1c-plasma lipids-creatinine-urine proteinuria-24 hr urine-ECG/oral and insulin/ophthalmology type1 within 5 yrs-type 2 immediately/HbA1c every 3 months-calibrate home glucose monitor-dip stick analysis of gross proteinuria-ECG-opthalmoscopy.
7. Rx complex carbohydrates—40 mt of exercise 4 days a week.
8. Blood glucose self monitoring-Type1-3 tests per day-if fasting FBG>14-ketone tests/if bedtime FBG<7-bedtime snack.
9. Total insulin required-Type 1-0.6U/kg/day (36 units for a 60 kg) and Type 2-0.3/kg/day (18 units for a 60 kg).
10. Rx life style changes for 2-4 months-if no change oral—Metformin or glyburide—ACE inhibitors for BP or kidney problems.

Diabetic ketoacidosis

Case: A 30 yr old patient with type I diabetes presents to the ER with abdominal pain and vomiting. Take H/o. Labs: Glucose 25, K 6.0, pH 7.22, Bicarb. 14. What is your diagnosis and management?

1. H/o for abdominal pain and vomiting: quality of pain, location, onset, chronology, radiation, associated symptoms, aggravating and relieving factors.
2. Number of episodes of vomiting, description of vomit, presence of blood and bile. Associated prodromal illness, fever, malaise, sore throat, cough, urinary symptoms, diarrhoea.
3. Foods eaten, other people sick? Previous similar episode?
4. Precipitants of DKA: Recent surgery, recent trauma, pregnancy.
5. Diabetes H/o: Time since diagnosis, medications, blood sugar monitor at home? Diabetic control, polyuria, polydipsia, diet, exercise, drugs, alcohol, smoking.
6. Complications of diabetes (retinopathy, neuropathy, nephropathy, infections).
7. Who follows patient's DM? Has patient taken insulin since feeling unwell? Last insulin dose?
8. PMH, other medications, allergies, family H/o, ROS.
9. Management: Foley, IV, lytes, glucose, ABG, serum ketones.
10. Septic work-up: CBC, CXR, blood cultures, urinalysis, ECG if K is critically elevated.
11. Rehydration—Bolus NS infusion until tachycardia and BP normalize.
12. Insulin initial bolus 5-10 IV in adults/followed by continuous infusion at 5-10 U per hour.
13. Add D5W when blood glucose is <15 mM
14. Replace potassium.
15. Check glucose and lytes q 2hr.
16. Begin diet and regular insulin regimen.
17. If the DKA was the result of non-compliance, close follow-up and education such as diet and diabetes management counselling with a dietician are required.

Bleeding disorder

Case: 30 yr old woman with 6 weeks of epistaxis, petechiae and easy bruising. Perform focussed P/E. Findings: petechiae, bruises. The patient has a normal CBC. Platelets 20 (normal 130-400). What is the most likely diagnosis? What four investigations would you order?

1. Patient undressed to underwear, draped below the waist.
2. Patient Sitting: Inspect for petechiae, abnormal skin tone, and hair falling out.
3. Inspect the finger and toe nails for dystrophy, flame hemorrhages, leukonychia.
4. Inspect the palm for erythema and Dupuytren's contractures.
5. Look in the nose and mouth for bleeding, petechiae, masses.
6. Palpate the anterior and posterior triangles of the neck, the supra and infra clavicular areas, and the axillae for lymph nodes.
7. Palpate the thyroid while standing behind the patient and patient swallows.
8. Chest—From behind the patient, inspect the skin. Percuss the lung fields for effusions and consolidations, auscultate the lung fields. Percuss and auscultate the anterior lung fields.
9. Listen over the aortic, pulmonary, tricuspid and mitral areas
10. Patient lying: Compress the sternum and ribcage for pain (multiple myeloma).
11. Inspect the abdomen. Auscultate for bowel sounds. Palpate for enlargement of the spleen and liver. Percuss the liver.
12. Palpate the groin for lymph nodes.
13. Note: Avoid rectal exam as this trauma may cause bleeding.
14. Most likely diagnosis: Idiopathic thrombocytopenic purpura (ITP).
15. 4 findings on H/o that help confirm the diagnosis: a. Remitting-relapsing course b. Mild fevers c. Splenic discomfort due to mild enlargement d. Bleeding after low doses of NSAID.
16. 4 investigations: Blood smear, INR/PTT (for hemophilia), serum urea/creatinine (for hemolytic-uremic syndrome), serum platelet-associated IgG (for ITP).

Counselling for high cholesterol

Dyslipidemia target lipid values are based on the risk factors—Major are smoking/DM/BP/hyperlipidemia/family h/o-minor obesity, sedentary, hyperhomocystinemia. The 10 year risk is calculated as follows. Note: points are given in brackets.

1. Age: 45-49—(3)/50-54 (6)/55-59 (8)/60-65 (10)/65-69 (11)/75-79 (13)
2. Total C: *Conversion rate from mmol/L to mgm%=38.7* e.g. 6.4 mmol/L=250 mgm%
    At age 40-49-> 5.14 (3)/6.2(4)/7.2(5)/>7.2 (8)
3. Smoking 40-49-(5)/50-59 (3)/60-69 (1)
4. HDL Below <1.24 to 1.04(1)/<1 (2)
5. Systolic BP >130 (1)/>160 (2)
    10   year   risk   in   %   based   on   points   added   up   are
    5(2%)/10(6%)/15(20%)/17(30%)

Lipid management: Higher the risk, greater the target. Now target lipid values are
    a. If <10% LDL <4.5 and Total C:HDL ratio <6
    b. If 11-19% LDL <3.5 and Total C:HDL ratio <5
    c. If >20 % LDL <2.5 and Total C: HDL ratio < 4

1. Also drug Rx after 3 months of diet treatment.
2. Rx with statins/bile acid sequestrants/nicotinic acid/fibrates/ezetimibe (cholesterol absorption inhibitor).
3. Estimate cholesterol after 1.5 and 3months/monitor ALT/CK/AST at baseline and at q 6 months to see myositis.
4. Lipid management: For cardiovascular disease and stroke:
5. Smoking/BP less than 140/90.
6. Diet/ASA/30 min of moderate exercise every week.
7. Weight: Keep a BMI between 18.5-24.9. If above 25 keep waist circ. less than 100 for male and less than 90 for females.
8. Diabetes management.
9. Chronic atrial fibrillation is converted to normal sinus rhythm or Rx with anticoagulation with INR 2 to 3/and the following.

Counseling to quit smoking

1. Elicit habits/previous quit attempts/results/need counseling sessions of 10 min each with 6-12 month follow up.
2. 4As to be done if willing to quit-Advise to quit/Assess willingness to quit/Assist/Arrange follow up.
3. Pregnant need to quit without nicotine replacement therapy (NRT). NRT has odds of quitting 1.5 to 2 regardless of additional support system.
4. No difference in methods of quitting. Effectiveness 20% compared to 10% with placebo.
5. Benefits: Reduce cravings-harmful substances in nicotine.
6. Side effects: Immediate post MI-angina worsens-arrythmias.
7. Antidepressant Bupropion inhibit re-uptake of dopamine/NA Rx for 6 months-patient continue to smoke for 2 weeks then stops/can be used with NRT/side effect dry mouth and insomnia.
8. Gum and patch are available in Canada. Gum-2 mgm if < 25 cigarettes-1 piece every 1-2 hours (24 pieces max a day). Chew until peppery and then park between gum and cheek for absorption. Continue chew and park for 30 min.
9. Nicotine patch: Use for 8 weeks—21mgX 4 weeks-14 mgm-2weeks-7 mgm-2 weeks-start low dose if <10 cigarettes-rotate with gum.
10. Explain the risks: SOB-asthma exacerbations-impotence-infertility-pregnancy complications—MI-stroke—COPD-lung CA-high risk for spousal and child lung CA-SIDS-asthma.
11. Benefits: Better food taste-good example to children.
12. Side effects: Wt gain-lack of support-fear of withdrawal.
13. If unsuccessful tell—Many people try and fail many times before success. Highest relapse during the first 3 months.
14. Congratulate on success. Encourage ongoing abstinence-review-negative mood-withdrawal-lack of support etc.

Obesity counsel

1. Body mass index = Weight in kilograms/Height in meters ^{2}
2. Waist circumference->102 cm in men and 88 cm in females assoc with risk factors-DM, BP, dyslipidemia, HTN, osteoarthritis,
3. Gall stone and CVS diseases.
4. Obesity = BMI >30—sleep apnea, osteoarthritis, smoking, CAD.
5. Assess motivation/weight loss recommended if BMI>30 or 25-29+2 risk factors.
6. Reducing 500-1000 kcal/day or 300-500 (if overweight) will cause wt loss nearly 1kg/week.
7. Do not eat while watching TV
8. Rx-Orlistat—Reduce GI fat absorption/Ezetimibe-Cholesterol absorption inhibitor/If >40 stomach stapling.

Section 4

Emergency Medicine

1. ECG

1. Rt. or Lt. atrial enlargement: Look at lead II
2. Rt. or Lt ventricular enlargement: Look at chest leads 1 to 6
3. MI—Acute (days) ST elevation/Recent (weeks to months) T wave inversion/Old (months to years) Just significant Qs.
4. Hyperkalemia—peaked T, flat P, wide QRS, long PR, elevated ST
5. Hypokalemia—flat T, U wave, ST depression, prolonged QT
6. Pericarditis—ST elevation in all leads
7. Heart block
   1st degree—PR more than 5 units (0.2 sec) No Rx
   2nd degree
     a. type 1. Progressive prolongation with missing. No Rx if no symptoms.
     b. type 2. QRS are dropped at regular intervals. PR is stable (normal or prolonged). Rx—pacemaker.
   3rd degree—No relation between P and QRS waves. Rate 30-60
   Rx—pacemaker.

2. Dead patient = VF or Pulseless VT

ABC,
O_2, IV, monitor

Defibrillate—100, 200, 300, 360 J. (Try 100J first, If fail go to the next and so on). The defibrillator is in asynchronous mode (given when there is no pulse). Give 100 J first. Say "I am going to defibrillate upon 3. One—I clear; Two—You clear;
3—Everyone clear".
Epinephrine 1 mgm every 5 mts (give until I say to stop)
Shock 360J
Amiodarone 300 mgm IV push
Shock 360 J
Amiodarone 150 mgm IV push
Rpt Shock 360 J and Amiodarone 150 mgm until pulse comes back and ECG rhythm turns to normal.

3. VT

If stable with pulse—Amiodarone 150 mgm IV over 10 mts.
Repeat every 10 mts (540 mgm over 18 hrs) as needed.
If not changing—synchronized cardioversion—100, 200, 300, 360 J

4. PSVT

Check for carotid bruit first. Carotid massage on one side
If not reversed—IV adenosine 6 mgm over 3 sec. followed by normal saline 20 ml bolus. Repeat max. 3 doses.
If not reversed—100 J synchronized.

5. Atrial Fibrillation

Less than 48 hrs—IV Amiodarone—150 mgm
More than 48 hrs—Diltiazem 20 mgm IV over 2 mts. Repeat in 15 mts.
Maintain 10 mgm/hour titrated to heart rate.

6. Atrial Flutter

Best is DC conversion 50 J

7. Tachycardia (unstable)

Unstable is when there is CCF, diastolic BP less than 80 mm Hg, pulse more than 150/min, chest pain and shortness of breath.

ABC, Oxygen, IV and monitor.

If conscious-premeditate with Fentanyl 2 microgm/mt (analgesia) and atropine 0.5 mgm and wait for 3 min.

For VT, PSVT and AF give 100, 200, 300, 360 J; For atrial flutter—50 J

8. Asystole

Check connections—Power switch, battery

ABC, Oxygen, IV fluids, monitor

CPR

If you see the asystole—Precordial thrust

Transcutaneous pacing (pads on the left side of the chest one on the anterior and another on the posterior side)

Epinephrine 1mgm IV repeat every 5 min (no max. limit)

Atropine 1 mgm IV push (3 doses max)

(Need long resuscitation for drug overdose)

9. Pulseless Electrical Activity

ABC, CPR, IV fluids, monitor

Epinephrine1mgm IV repeat every 5 min (no max. limit)

Atropine1 mgm IV push (3 doses max)

Treatable causes

   a)   hypovolemia, hypokalemia, hyperkalemia, hypoxia, hypothermia, Hydrogen ion (acidity)

   b)   Tablets, tamponade, tension pneumothorax, thrombosis (coronary, pulmonary)

10. Bradycardia

Less than 60/min. Not an emergency

ABC, Oxygen, IV fluids, Monitor

Symptomatic—Transcutneous pacing (pads on the left side of the chest one on the anterior and another on the posterior side)

Atropine-0.5 mgm IV (Atropine 1mgm if dead; 0.5 mgm if alive)

Epinephrine 1mgm IV

Dopamine 5-20 microgram/kg/min

11. Myocardial infarction

ABC, Oxygen, IV fluids, Monitor, 12 lead ECG
(MONA greets them all—Morphine, Oxygen, Nitrites, Aspirin)
Morphine 2-5 mgm IV q 5-30 min.
Oxygen
Nitroglycerin 0.3 mgm sublingual x 3
Aspirin 2 baby or 325 mgm tab to chew
Severe chest pain—IV Beta blockers, tPA-15 mgm IV bolus, 40mgm next 30 min, 30 mgm next 60 min, and low molecular weight heparin 1mg/kg S.C bid.
If BP—Metoprolol 5 mgm IV q 5 min x 3 (not in inferior wall MI).
Thrombolytics indications
a. ST elevation >1mm in 2 or more contiguous leads
b. If you see the patient within 12 hours
c. LBBB
d. With a duration of 30 min of pain
Trombolytics contraindications
a. Dissecting aneurysm
b. Active bleeding
c. Haemorragic shock
d. Pericarditis
PCI (Percutaneous coronary intervention) indications

If no ECG changes but if cardiac enzymes ++
Aspirin, 2b 3a inhibitors, unfragmented heparin, beta blockers IV
ST depression MI
Aspirin, 2b 3a inhibitors, unfragmented heparin, beta blockers IV + Heparin
Arrythmias
Antiarrythics, cardioversion/defibrillation.

12. Heart blocks

1st degree—PR more than 5 units (0.2 sec) No Rx
2nd degree Type 1. Progressive prolongation with missing of PR. No Rx if no symptoms.

2nd degree Type 2. QRS are dropped at regular intervals. PR is stable (normal or prolonged). Rx-pacemaker.

3rd degree—No relation between P and QRS waves. Distance between Ps is same. Distance between QRS is same. Rx—pacemaker.
Note: First give trans-cutaneous pacing. Then can go for trans-venous pacing and later elective permanent pacemaker.

13. Miscellaneous

Atypical presentations—By females, DM, old age, Indians
Inferior wall MI (leads 2, 3, AVF)—ask for a 15 lead ECG—because right coronary artery supplies both inferior and right side.
If right sided MI is diagnosed—Give IV fluids to increase the fluid load.

14. Stable angina

Rx. Beta blockers (first line).
Ca channel blockers—Second line or combination with ACE inhibitors
Nitrates/Life style changes/ECASA
Nitrates—Short acting.
Lipid lowering agents.
Percutaneous Coronary Intervention (PCI)
CABG-indicated in all unstable and stable with left main/3 vessel/4 vessel.

15. Congestive cardiac failure

Rx: ABC
Sit upright
IV TKVO only.
100% oxygen
0.3mg nitro S/L q 5min PRN
Frusomide 4-80 mgm IV
Morphine 1-2 mgm IV
Dopamine 5-10 microgm/kg/min IV if hypotensive
ASA 160 mgm chew
Treat any infection

Chest Pain

Case: 57 year old man comes with right sided chest pain and mild breathing difficulty.

- Identify yourself as the team leader by saying "I am the team leader"
- Say " I am wearing gloves, gown and mask"
- ABC—(A-look at mouth and feel chest expansion, trachea.
  B-listen at mouth, auscultate trachea andchest. C-peripheral pulse, heart sound and JVP. Always tell what you are looking for or doing.
- 100 % oxygen by mask
- Two 14 gauge peripheral IV lines with 2 L Ringer lactate run wide open (depending on the amount of bleeding)
- Vitals please
- Hook up pulse oximeter (Oxygen saturation)
- EKG, Continuous cardiac monitor
- Cervical spine collar
- X-ray AP chest, pelvis, lateral spine
- Warming blanket
- Send blood for "CBC, lytes, urea, creatinine, LFT, RFT, PT, PTT, INR, blood gases, glucose, lactate, amylase, Ca, Mg, phosphate"
- Blood group, screen, cross match for 6 units of packed RBCs
- ABC
- Vitals please
- AVPU—Alert, responds to verbal stimuli, responds to pain, unresponsive
- Log roll the patient and palpate the spine
- ABC
- Vitals please
- Secondary survey—take a H/o (either from the patient or from the nurse)
- Examine head, neck, eyes, ears, nose, skull, chest, abdomen, rectal exam, pelvic stability, musculoskeletal exam, neurological exam (reflexes and tone).
- Nasogastric tube, Foley's catheter, abdominal USG, diagnostic peritoneal lavage.
- CT—chest, abdomen and pelvis
- General surgery consultation
- Reduced BP, distended neck veins, muffled heart sound—pericardial tamponade—pericardiocentesis.
- Reduced BP, hypoxia and dull chest—haemothorax—IV fluid, blood, decompress—intercostals drain through 5th space mid axillary line and under water seal.
- Resonant on percussion, trachea shift to one side—pneumothorax—14 gauge angiocath needle—2nd intercostal space, midclavicular line.

Hemoptysis

Case: 60 yr old male with hemoptysis and SOB. Take H/o.

1. H/o of CAD, HTN, hasn't been taking antihypertensives for 6 weeks.
2. Onset of symptoms, duration, time of day. Has patient had these before?
3. Smoking H/o, fatigue, ankle edema, orthopnea, PND, palpitations, chest pain/heaviness/tightness, pain in left arm or jaw/teeth.
4. H/o of angina or other cardiac problems.
5. H/o of GI bleeds, reflux, varices, gastritis, peptic ulcer. COPD H/o, cough, sputum, wheeze.
6. H/o of immobilization, leg pain or swelling, previous DVT, PE. Medications—has patient been taking them?
7. Drugs, alcohol, allergies, surgical H/o, family H/o, ROS.
8. CXR shows enlarged heart, upper lobe vascular redistribution, Kerley B lines, bilateral interstitial infiltrates and bilateral small effusions. CXR: Consistent with pulmonary edema and CHF.
9. ECG: Shows Q waves and inverted T waves in V1-4.
10. What is the diagnosis? Anterior wall MI.

Coma

Case: 79 yr old woman collapses in the mall. Patient is drowsy, unresponsive to verbal stimuli. Manage. Findings: HR 40, BP: 80/40, ECG: complete heart block.

1. "Unstable" means either an acutely changing condition, vital signs dangerously beyond normal ranges (e.g. Low BP).
2. This patient is unstable due to dangerous hypotension, has an acutely changing condition and therefore requires stabilization or resuscitation.
3. Manage according to the ACLS and ATLS formats.
4. Primary survey: ABCD
5. Airway: Check for patient airway (look in mouth), is airway threatened by blood?
6. High chance of aspiration due to poor level of consciousness, neck or face swelling.
7. If airway is compromised, immediately place an oral airway or incubate.
8. Breathing: Is patient breathing, check O_2 sat may require immediate manual bag-valve mask followed by intubations with positive pressure ventilation.
9. Circulation: BP, HR, rhythm on monitor, active high volume bleeding.
10. Patient may require immediate chest compressions or defibrillation.
11. Glasgow coma scale (GCS):

	Eye opening	Verbal	Motor
6			obeys
5		oriented	localizes to pain
4	spontaneous	confused	withdraws to pain
3	to speech	inappropriate words	decorticate posture
2	to pain	sounds	decerebrate posture
1	none	none	no movement

12. Standard painful stimulus is rubbing the knuckle on the sternum.
13. For withdrawal, apply pressure on the base of the nail bed with a pen.
14. Decorticate posture is arm flexion with leg extension on the same side of the body, may be unilateral or bilateral. Indicates a lesion above the brainstem.
15. Decerebrate posture is arm and ipsilateral leg extension, may be unilateral or bilateral. Indicates brainstem involvement.

16. A GCS of 8 or less is considered an indication for intubations because of the risk of poor protection of the airway from aspiration.
17. Primary Orders: Oxygen, monitoring (cardiac, O_2 sat, automatic BP cuff or arterial line), IV access: need 2 large-bore lines (16 gauge, 14 if possible) run wide open with normal saline for acutely low BP, may need to be more restrained if pulmonary edema is a problem.
18. Coma cocktail if diagnosis not known already: Thiamine 100 mg IV, narcan 1 mg IV, flumazenil 0.1 mg IV (1 amp D50 is no longer included in this cocktail because of deleterious effects of high serum glucose on the injured brain).
19. Initial investigations: CBC, lytes, urea, Cr, ABG, glucose, ionized Ca, CK-MB, INR/PTT, ECG, portable CXR, cross-table lateral C-spine and hard collar if there is a head injury or any significant trauma.
20. Secondary Survey: Head to tow P/E. Vitals. Head and Neck: inspect for lacerations and contusions, pupillary response, doll's eyes (careful of neck—may not be able to turn head enough to do this), corneal reflexes, palpate facial bones for stability, look in nose and ears for blood or CSF leaks, hemotympanum.
21. Check oral cavity, gag reflex, palpate dorsal cervical spines for pain and alignment, is the trachea midline?
22. Chest: breath sounds, heart sounds, radial pulses bilaterally.
23. Abdomen: Rigidity is an indicator for immediate general surgery, auscultate for bowel sounds, palpate liver and spleen.
24. Log roll patient onto back, inspect, palpate the spine. Palpate for pelvic stability and intactness of long bones, PR examination.
25. Secondary Orders: Foley, nasogastric tube if patient may go to surgery or require charcoal. Specific interventions based on findings.
26. Further X-rays, CT head if cause of decreased consciousness unclear or if there may have been a seizure.
27. Clearing C-spine: The principle of clearing C-spines is to rule out both fractures and ligamentous injury, either of which can make the spine dangerously unstable. May clear cervical spine in the case of an alert patient who has no pain on palpation of the dorsal spinous processes and a normal cross-table lateral C-spine x-ray.
28. If the patient has neck pain, flexion/extension plane films are done.
29. Flexion/extension views may be done under fluoroscopy if the patient is not alert.
30. H/o: If available. Nature of collapse, preceding and subsequent events, has patient ever experienced similar symptoms before, did patient lose consciousness, were there seizure-type phenomena, injuries during the fall, duration of unconsciousness, post ictal drowsiness, medications and drugs, smoking, allergies, PMH, family H/o, ROS.

31. Management of complete heart block: (P waves seen on ECG not related to QRS complexes) Transcutaneous pacing (Atropine 1 mg IV may be tried but is rarely effective), patient will require sedation (midazolam 2 mg IV) and analgesia (morphine 2 mg IV) before starting external pacing.
32. Will require placement of a transvenous pacer until a permanent pacer can be placed. Consult Cardiology/CCU/ICU.
33. Causes of AV conduction abnormalities: Calcification of the conducting system, inferior MI, coronary spasm, digitalis overdose, TCA overdose, beta blockers, calcium channel blockers, viral infection, rheumatic fever, Lyme disease, sarcoid, amyloidosis, hemochromatosis, cardiac tumour, congenital.

Case: 42 yr old man found unconscious in the street. Appears that he was struck on the head. Perform P/E. Findings: GCS 11, unilateral body weakness. What is your DDx? Evaluate C-spine film. Describe your initial treatment and investigations.

1. Resuscitate.
2. P/E: should include a neurological exam.
3. GCS, if patient unresponsive apply deep pain stimulation using sternal rub to elicit posturing.
4. Mental status.
5. cranial nerves: Extra-ocular eye movements, visual fields by confrontation, pupillary reactivity and accomodation, corneal reflex and facial sensation, facial muscle power, gross hearing, gag, sternocleidomastoid power and trapezius power.
6. Pronator drift, cerebellar tests: finger-nose, heel shin, rapid alternating movements (dysdiadokinesis).
7. Muscle power, tone, sensation.
8. Deep tendon reflexes, Babinski's test.
9. DDx: concussion, subdural bleed, epidural bleed, brain contusion, seizure or post-ictal weakness, brainstem or spinal cord injury.
10. C-spine film evaluation.
11. Treatment: Normalize vitals, O_2 saturation, ABGs, hydrate to maintain BP, give blood if necessary, correct coagulopathy, and immobilize C-spine.
12. Consider intubation (careful about the neck).
13. Control ICP: Load with Dilantin 1 g IV to prevent seizures, give 20% mannitol 50 g IV, rapid sequence intubation with lidocaine and hyperventilate to pCO_2 35.
14. Consult neurosurgery.
15. CT head and neck.
16. May need MRI for identification of brainstem or spinal cord injuries.

Drug overdose

Case: 25 year old male with tricyclic antidepressant overdose. Manage.

Resuscitation—ABC.
Take H/o from the patient/family member/friend.
Ask for the empty pill bottles to confirm the drug.
How many pills? When was it taken?
Ingestions of alcohol or other drugs?
Where was the patient found?
Was there a period of unconsciousness? How long did this last?
Blurring of vision, seizure?
Did the patient give any warning (note, phone calls, giving away possessions)?
Was there a preceding depression or strange behaviour?
Problems at work or relationship?
Previous attempts?
Medications, drugs, alcoholism, smoking, allergies, PMH, psychiatric H/o, family H/o.
Investigations: CBC, lytes, urea, Cr, glucose, INR/PTT, ABG, CK, serum osmolality, Alk Phos, AST, ALT, total bilirubin, GGT, Tox. screen—ASA, acetaminophen, TCA levels, ECG, CXR (for aspiration pneumonia).

Treatment: Gastric lavage within 1 hour of ingestion.
Activated charcoal 10 g by nasogastric tube.
Hydrate with NS to promote diuresis for excretion of TCA and myoglobin.
Alkalinize with 1 amp bicarb IV (or 1-2 mEq/kg)
Follow ABGs or venous gases, aim for pH 7.45—7.55.
Treat seizures with lorazepam 2 mg IV,
Treat cardiac dysrhythmias, hypotension, agitation.
Consult ICU for 24 hours for monitoring.
Psychiatric consult after patient is medically cleared.

TCA toxicity: Therapeutic level 2-4 mg/kg. Life threatening levels >10 mg/kg.
"Hot as a hare, Blind as a bat, Dry as a bone, Red as a beet, Mad as a hatter".
Anti-cholinergic effects: hyperthermia, tachycardia, dilated pupils, decreased sweating and secretions, vasodilation, constipation, urinary retention, ileus.
CNS effects: Generalized seizures, myoclonus, ataxia, hyper-reflexia, confusion, agitation, hallucinations, acute psychosis, decreased consciousness, respiratory depression.

<u>Quinidine effects:</u> Conduction delay (prolonged QRS, PR, QT, T-wave flattening), heart block, bradycardia, asystole, ventricular dysrhythmias and hypotension.

Case: 16 yr old female in hospital for ASA overdose. Medically cleared. Take H/o.

1.   H/o: Patient name, age, occupation.
2.   Circumstances surrounding the attempted suicide.
3.   Preceding conflicts at work or with family or in a relationship.
4.   Recent loss of employment or loved one. Warning signs: Suicide note, giving away possessions.
5.   Describe the attempt, how many pills taken, what kinds, concurrent alcohol or drug use.
6.   Did the patient really want to die or was the attempt a cry for help?
7.   Gauge the lethality of the attempt in terms of the means used and the chances of discovery.
8.   Previous attempts, describe these. Is patient now actively suicidal or remorseful?
9.   If the patient is actively suicidal, what is the current plan?
10. Depression H/o and MMSE. Medications, drug/alcohol use, allergies, PMH, family H/o (esp. psychiatric), social supports, ROS.

Section 5

Geriatrics

Falls

Case 1: 76 yr. old woman brought in your office because of repeated falls.
Case 2: You are in to assess a 70 yrs. old man who just fell in his house.
Case 3: You are called to see a 78 years old man in the clinical ward because he fell after trying to walk around.

1. First of all make sure that the patient is ok.
2. OCD
3. Ask about injuries, dizziness,
4. Ask how many times this happened (recurrent falls= >2 in a 6 month-period); When was the last time?
5. Where did it happen? = home (bathroom, kitchen, living room, escalators, basement)
6. Analyze the episode. Any witness?
7. Before the fall: Dizziness, lightheadedness, vertigo, headaches, CP, SOB, palpitations, weakness, hunger, visual disturbance, fever.
8. Did you slip, skip?
9. During: Did you hurt yourself? LOC? seizure? bleeding? diarrhea?
10. After: Headache, pain, confusion, loc, timing to recover?
11. You should be able to recognize if the fall was related to: syncope, vertigo, environmental hazards, acute illness, epilepsy, and stroke.
12. Risk factors:
    a. Extrinsic: Environmental hazards: poor light, carpets, furniture, stairs, irregular floor,
    b. Intrinsic:Acute/chronic diseases: older >75 years, living alone, using cane/walker, cognitive impairment
13. Medications, (particularly if combination >4 or new medications incorporate in the last 2 weeks)
14. Reduced vision, foot problems, decreased hearing.
15. Tremor, rigidity, akinesia, postural change.
16. Anemia: fatigue, if B12 deficiency look for neurological symptoms.
17. Hypothyroidism: Fatigue, edemas, cold intolerance, confusion, weight gain.
18. Depression: Sadness, insomnia, weight loss, isolation,
19. Stroke: Weakness, speech problems, memory problems,
20. Dementia: Forgetfulness, wrong word, non able to do ADL/IADL.
21. ADL (Activities of daily life)—DEATH = Dressing, Eating, Ambulating, Toileting, Hygiene.
22. IADLs (Instrumental activities of daily life)—SHAFT = Shopping, Housekeeping, Accounting, Food preparation, Transportation

23. OA: Joint pain, joint swelling, and limitation on movements.
24. PMH: DM, HTN, Parkinson's, OA, trauma, osteoporosis, heart diseases, bleeding, surgeries, depression, dementia, cancer.
25. Medications: Always ask sedative-hypnotics, anxiolytics, TCS, anti-hypertensives, cardiac medication (diuretics), steroids, NSAIDS, anticholinergics, hypoglycemics, polypharmacy increases the risk of falling.
26. Allergies, alcohol smoking, drugs,
27. Living alone? Widow/er?
28. Diet (tea and toast is frequent in elderly living alone or with dental problems), finances, drug plan, family relationship, abuse, change in environment.
29. Attitude towards life?
30. Address patient's concerns and expectations.

When you finish think if
   a. Is anything acute? Anything reversible?
   b. Can any medication be changed?
   c. Can physiotherapy help?
   d. Can any environmental or behavioral modification be made?
   e. Develop a home safety checklist to reduce the risk of falls
   f. Address RF for falls and osteoporosis and fractures in old age.

If you have to examine the patient:
1. Ask the vitals and look for orthostatic changes (Lie down—pulse, BP, make to sit down—wait for 1 minute—pulse, BP).
2. Inspection: look abnormal postures, tremors, asymmetries, facial expression, skin, nutritional status,
3. Head neck and ENT, thyroid.
4. Ask to get up and walk (analyze if the patient has problem getting up w/o help, also analyze gait,
5. Volume status.
6. CV exam (arrhythmias, valvular diseases)
7. Neuro exam: Particularly visual acuity, hearing tests, balance/equilibrium, signs of Parkinson, motor, sensorial, CNS, Romberg, sternal nudge test, posterior cord, cerebellum,
8. MSK: Signs of OA, muscle wasting, inflammation, leg-length discrepancy, foot problems.
9. Abdomen (also DRE looking malena if applies)
10. The MMSE should be included.

Case 1: Orthostatic hypotension secondary to medications
Case 2: Fall related to acute illness (pneumonia)
Case 3: Fall related to acute delirium

DVT

Case: 60 yr old male slipped and fell 6 days ago. Visits due to hemoptysis. Perform a focussed P/E. Finding: Positive Homan's sign. What is the most likely diagnosis? Give a plan for management.

a. P/E plus additional attention to calf size, tenderness, redness, and pleuritic chest pain. Homan's sign: pain in the calf on dorsiflexion of the foot—indicates thrombophlebitis.
b. Check that trachea is midline.
c. Is the patient on DVT prophylaxis or anti-coagulation?
d. Most Likely Dx: Pulmonary embolus.
e. Specific Investigations for PE: CT chest (only shows clinically significant PE), V/Q scan (conclusive when it shows high or low probability), and serial (q 2 days) leg Dopplers for presence of DVT above the knee.
f. Treatment: If suspicion of PE is high, anticoagulate before waiting for these tests with heparin 7500 units IV bolus (80 units/kg), then infuse at 1200 units/hr (18 units/kg). Measure PTT q 6hr, adjust dose for PTT 70-90 seconds (2.5 to 3 x normal baseline). Start coumadin to get an INR of 2-3, continue coumadin for 3 months.

Case: Elderly woman in hospital pot-op day 5 of total hip replacement. Acute chest pain, tachycardia, and shortness of breath. Manage.

1. Life-threatening causes of acute chest pain: MI, PE, pneumothorax and tension pneumothorax, aortic dissection.
2. Other causes: Angina, gastritis, reflux, peptic ulcer, pericarditis, herpes zoster, MSK.
3. Rapid cardiopulmonary H/o including any H/o of high blood pressure, heart problems, smoking, COPD.
4. P/E plus additional attention to calf size, tenderness, redness and pleuritic chest pain.
5. Homan's Sign: Pain in the calf on dorsiflexion of the foot—indicates thrombophlebitis.
6. Check that trachea is midline. Inspect the surgical wound. Is the patient on DVT prophylaxis or anti-coagulation?
7. Treatment: Raise head of bed. Give oxygen 6L/min by mask. Monitor oxygen saturation (order stat CBC, lytes, glucose, INR/PTT, CK-MB, ABG, CXR, ECG).
8. Give chewable ASA 160-325 mg immediately.

9. Secure IV access, bolus IV lasix 40 mg push if fluid overload is suspected, and ventolin if wheezes are heard, give sublingual nitro spray or 0.3 mg sublingual nitroglycerin if blood pressure is adequate and 1 mg morphine IV.

10. Repeat nitroglycerin q 5 min X 3.

11. May require additional morphine and nitroglycerin.

12. Repeat CK-MB q 8hr x 3. ECG: If ECG shows significant ST elevation (more than 1mm in two anatomically consecutive leads), or a new left bundle branch block, then the patient is having an MI.

13. Order immediate cardiology consultation for possible lytic therapy or cardiac catheterization.

14. If less severe signs of ischemia are present (flipped T waves, ST depression), follow with repeat ECGs until resolved. S1Q3T3: This classic pattern (wide S-wave in lead 1, Q-waves in lead III, T wave inversion in lead III) with right axis deviation and RBBB are signs of right heart strain seen in massive PE.

15. An elevated A-a (alveolar pO_2-arterial pO_2) gradient is a sign of pulmonary embolus; but also occurs in conditions with a ventilation-perfusion mismatch (e.g. Pneumonia, PE, COPD). It is calculated from the ABG: A-a = $713(FiO_2)$—$1.25(PaCO_2)$-PaO_2 (normal 12 in child, 20 in 70 yr old). Note that the inspired oxygen fraction (FiO_2) is not known unless the patient is on room air, a ventimask, or mechanically ventilated. This is because the patient breathes in more by an unknown amount than the output of nasal prongs or ordinary mask. Roughly, however, 2L/min gives 26% FiO_2, 3L=30%, 4L=35%, and 6L=40%. 40% is considered the maximum inspired oxygen obtainable without a high flow mask such as a ventimask.

16. ABG normal values: pH 7.35-7.45, pO_2 80-100 mmHg, bicarb 24, pCO_2 40 Indications for intubation: An ABG showing poor pO_2 (in the 60s or if less than 80 on high inspired oxygen concentrations), elevated pCO_2 (greater than 80), acidemia, or GCS<8 (not able to protect airway) may indicate need for intubation if these are not quickly correctable. Consult ICU.

17. CXR sign of PE: Wedge-shaped infiltrate (Hampton's hump) or oligemic area, unilateral effusion, raised hemidiaphragm.

18. A normal CXR is also consistent, and usual, with PE.

19. Specific Investigations for PE: CT chest (can only see PE which is large enough to be clinically significant), V/Q scan (conclusive when it shows high or low probability), and serial (q 2 days) leg Dopplers for presence of DVT above the knee.

20. Treatment/: If suspicion of PE is high, anticoagulate before waiting for tests with heparin 7500 units IV bolus, then infuse at 1200 units/hr, Measure PTT q 6hr, adjust dose for PTT 70-90 sec.

21. If a diagnosis of PE is made, give warfarin, continue anti-coagulation for 3 months.

Anaemia

Case: 65 yr old man with ataxia, dizziness, macrocytic anemia. Take H/o. Finding: Poor diet. Give a DDx. What is the most likely diagnosis? What investigations would you order?

1.   Onset, chronology, description of symptoms.
2.   Setting in which symptoms occur.
3.   Functional limitations (driving, walking, stairs, reaching upwards).
4.   Differentiate light-headedness from true vertigo (room or self-spinning).
5.   Peripheral numbness, psychiatric features: mild depression, irritability, paranoia (seen in B12 deficiency).
6.   Weakness, eye symptoms, tremor.
7.   TIA or stroke phenomena: Sudden neurological deficit (loss of vision, speech, motor or sensory changes).
8.   Check for heart problems, hypertension, diabetes.
9.   CAGE alcoholism screen.
10. H/o of syphilis, MS, hypothyroidism (decreases secretion of intrinsic factor), use of chemotherapeutic agents (interfere with DNA synthesis).
11. Diet, weight loss or gain, chronic diarrhea (malabsorption), abdominal pain.
12. Signs of intracranial hypertension (hydrocephalus): morning nausea, vomiting, headache.
13. General signs of malignancy: anorexia, fatigue, night sweats. PMH, medications, drugs/alcohol, smoking, allergies, family H/o, ROS.
14. DDx: anemia due to vitamin deficiency of B12 or folate (B6) usually due to malabsorption (lack of intrinsic factor—pernicious anemia, long term use of antacids, pancreatic insufficiency) or malnutrition (vegan diet). Severe hypothyroidism.
15. Medication or drug-induced, Wernicke's encephalopathy, hepatic encephalopathy, inner ear problem (BPV, acoustic neuroma, Meniere's), postural hypotension, brainstem stroke or TIA, intracranial tumour.
16. Most Likely Dx: Pernicious anemia
17. Investigations: CBC with blood smear, lytes, urea, Cr, INR/PTT, GGT, AST, ALT, Alk. Phos., serum folate, screen for serum B12, serum ferritin, Schilling's test: measures absorption of B12.
18. Barium enema (pernicious anemia is associated with bowel cancers).

Multiple Pains

Case: 60 yr old woman with multiple pains. Investigated by several other doctors, all lab tests were normal. Manage

1. Depression with somatization: Major depression presents with a somatic complaint, commonly headache, stomach pains, sleep disturbance, eating disturbance, or bowel habit changes. This is a frequent presentation of depression in the elderly.
2. Somatization disorder: Multiple non-intentional complaints in multiple organ systems beginning before age 30 that occur over several years, with treatment sought and significant impairment in functioning. Diagnostic criteria: 4 pain symptoms at 4 different sites, 2 GI symptoms other than pain, one reproductive or sexual symptom other than pain, one pseudo-neurological symptom (temporary blindness).
3. Conversion disorder: Psychic perturbation presents as one or two neurological complaints.
4. Chronic post-traumatic or post-surgical pain. Pain not fully accounted for by current tissue injury, exacerbated by psychic factors and associated with functional impairment.
5. Hypochondriasis: Exaggeration or misinterpretation of normal physiological features to the point of functional disability. Associated with obsessive fear of serious illness and doctor shopping.
6. Fibromyalgia: 80-90% of cases occur in middle-aged women, may afflict 5% of adult women. Associated with absent or decreased non-REM stage of sleep. Wake from sleep feeling unrefreshed. Constant, aching, axial pain with bilateral tender points (not trigger points where pain is triggered due to myofascial pain from overuse, e.g. tennis elbow). The disorder follows a waxing and waning course without progression or resolution and may become disabling. Characteristic reproducible tender points are located bilaterally at lateral border of sternum, sternocleidomastoid, posterior neck, trapezius, rhomboids, over sacroiliac joints, lateral thigh, posterior and medial knee. Patient should have 11 of the above 18 tender points for a diagnosis.
7. Chronic Fatigue Syndrome: Similar to fibromyalgia but fatigue is the dominant feature and pain and tender points may be less prominent or absent.
8. Factitious disorder or Malingering: Factitious disorder involves misrepresentation of history and symptoms for the purpose of assuming the sick role for secondary gains (attention and sympathy, justification for inadequacies).

9. Munchausen's syndrome is a type of factitious disorder in which P/E findings are faked by contamination of lab tests or ingestion of inappropriate medications or substances. Typically, the patient is a medical staff motivated by hostility toward health care set up. e. g. takes coumadin to fake hemophilia.

10. Malingering is distinguished from factitious disorder by a motivation for secondary gain other than the sick role. e.g. insurance benefits.

a. Pain description, location, duration, chronology, aggravating and relieving factors, are pains linked to one another?

b. Somatoform disorders screen: How has your health been for most of your life?

c. How have your pains affected your job, social life, relationships, and your life generally?

d. Are you often unwell? Do you often visit the doctor?

e. Do you worry that you have a serious illness?

f. If a doctor tells you that there is nothing medically wrong, how does that make you feel? Do you believe him or her?

g. Associated symptoms: Review of systems, medications, allergies, smoking, alcohol, drug use, family H/o.

h. Take depression H/o. Diagnosis and treatment: For non-specific pains with depressive symptoms, the patient most likely has depression with somatization. Rx for depression.

i. Rx: Counselling.

Confusion

Case: 60 yr old woman with acute confusion. Perform a focussed P/E excluding mental status

1. Neurologic Exam: Done with patient sitting, then standing, then lying down positions.
2. Every P/E should include vitals, although examiner (or SP) will ask to move on.
3. <u>Patient sitting</u>: GCS only if patient poorly responsive. Examiner will remind you to omit the MMSE.
4. Cranial nerves. Extra-ocular movements (patient follows your finger or the handle of a reflex hammer in an "H" pattern, check for diplopia in the centre and at the extremities of the visual fields.
5. Pupillary light reflex and accommodation, corneal reflex. Fundi, checking for papilloedema using ophthalmoscope.
6. Facial sensation to light touch in the ophthalmic, maxillary, and mandibular divisions of the trigeminal nerve. Facial muscle power—"raise eyebrows, keep eyes closed, show teeth, protrude tongue, observe palatal movement on saying "Ah""
7. Gag reflex: Observe symmetric movement of the palate.
8. Hearing: rub thumb and finger together while approaching the patient's ear, note when they can hear the sound.
9. Sternocleidomastoid power and trapezius power.
10. Hoffman's reflex: With the patient's relaxed hand in a palm-down position, squeeze and flick the nail of the index finger between your thumb and long finger. Thumb flexion indicates a +ive test and denotes upper motor neuron lesion (similar to Babinski's reflex).
11. Palmomental reflex—scratch palm and twitch of ipsilateral mentalis/orbicularis oris.
12. Cerebellar tests: finger-nose, rapid alternating movements (dysdiadocokinesis).
13. Muscle power: Deltoids, triceps, wrist extension and flexion, finger abduction and adduction, psoas (hip flexion of each knee off the bed against resistance), quadriceps, hamstrings, ankle dorsiflexion (test plantar flexion while standing).
14. Body sensation: Light tough, pin prick, cold temperature (use metal—tuning fork)—test on the distal upper limbs (forearms and hands) and lower limbs (foreleg and feet). Vibration sensation is tested using a 120 Hz tuning fork on the bony projections of the most distal joints.

15. Reflexes: Biceps, triceps, brachioradialis, knee, ankle, Babinski.
16. <u>Patient standing</u>: Gait—observe for wide-base, Parkinson's shuffle, lateralizing falls.
17. Balance: Rhomberg—feet together, eyes closed.
18. Hold patient's hands for balance, ask patient to stand on one foot, then raise themselves up on their toes.
19. <u>Patient lying</u>: Tone—passive rapid alternating forearm rotation, passive rapid elbow flexion/extension with one thumb on the biceps tendon to feel for cogwheel rigidity. Rapid lifting of the relaxed leg from behind the knee—normally heel remains on the bed.

Section 6

Pediatrics

Jaundice
Vomiting
Diarrhea
Pallor
Cough
Abdominal pain
Failure to thrive and neglect
Enuresis
Hyperactive child
Fever
Seizure
Meningitis
Child abuse
Dysuria
Asthma
Not speaking
Immunization
Alcoholism counsel
Feeding/diet counseling
Breast milk counseling

Note: Most of the time pediatric patients won't be there. Parent will be there to talk with. Usually the situation is that the child is in the emergency room next to you or the child is at home. Always ask about the child. Call the child by "Little Tom/Nancy/etc"

Jaundice

Case1: You are going to see Mrs. X on the obstetrical ward because her 4 day old baby is jaundiced. Take the H/o and address her questions.
Case2: Mrs. X brings her 1 week old son for the first prenatal check up. She notices that her baby looks "yellow". Interview her.

1. Congratulate the mother. How the baby is doing?
2. In case 1, ask why she and the baby are still in the hospital?
3. Start asking about the jaundice: Onset, course, duration. First newborn
4. Associated symptoms: Does the bay look well? (4 H: hemolysis, hypothyroidism, hematomas, hepatitis).
    Hemolysis: Easy bruising, petechiae, seizures. Kernicterus: abnormal movements, abnormal posture, seizures, lethargic.
    Hypothyroid: Abnormal facial expression, macroglossia, unripe umbilical cord.
    Hematomas: Asymmetric head, trauma during delivery.
    Hepatitis: Vomiting/diarrhea, petechiae, distended abdomen, urine color.
    Sepsis: Alert, cranky, lethargic, floppy, sucking well, seizures, SOB, cyanosis, fever, vomiting, diarrhea.

5. Pre-natal: Gestational age at birth, blood group/type, was the mother given Rhogam? previous jaundiced babies? transfusions?
    TORCHES infections: Toxoplasmosis (from cats, infects foetal brain), Rubella (teratogenic), herpes (infects foetus, fatal), CMV (damages foetal liver).
    Drugs, alcohol, smoking, IUGR, DM (large baby), preclampsia, hypertension, polyhydramnios, genetic abnormalities, infections: hepatitis, HIV, teratogenic medications. Hyper/hypothyroid, hypercoagulation.
    Natal: Was the baby in distress? difficulty in delivery? trauma? caesarean induction, rupture of membranes—artificial or prolonged (PROM), chorioamnionitis, forceps or vacuum delivery, meconium, APGARs, was resuscitation required, initial blood work, breast feeding—how often and how well, colour of first stool, colour of urine, vomiting, neonate muscle tone, fever, irritability, lethargy.
    Post-natal: Weight, APGAR, resuscitation, meconium, congenital abnormalities, admitted in neonatal ICU, phototherapy, transfusions.
6. Risk factors: Prematurity, acidosis, sepsis, dehydration, hypoalbuminemia, gestational DM.
7. PMH: Diseases of relevance.

8. Medications and allergies.
9. Feeding H/o: Breast-feeding?
10. Family H/o: Ethnic background, bleeding disorders, liver problems, previous babies with neonatal jaundice.
11. Investigations: Direct (conjugated) and indirect (unconjugated) bilirubin, neonatal and maternal blood types, blood smear, CBC with reticulocyte count. Septic work-up. Urinalysis, blood cultures, CXR, CSF.
12. Direct Coomb's test: Detects presence of anti-red cell autoimmune antibodies attached to baby's RBCs.
13. Indirect Coomb's test: Detects presence of anti-red cell antibodies in mother's serum.
14. Severe hyperbilirubinemia may lead to kernicterus—deposition of bilirubin in the brainstem and basal ganglia and lead to mental retardation, cerebral palsy, hearing loss and paralysis of upward gaze.
15. Normal bilirubin is nearly 200μmol/L. Serum total bilirubin level >300μmol/L is an indication for phototherapy. Water soluble photoisomers of bilirubin are produced and excreted without conjugation with glucuronic acid (normally bilirubin needs to be conjugated to become water soluble for excretion).
16. Levels greater than 400μmol/L—Exchange transfusion (replaces the baby's blood with donor blood) or plasmaphoresis (replace blood plasma with donor plasma)
17 D/d: Physiological jaundice: On day 2-3 in 50% of term infants. Often in pre-term infants where it manifests even up to day 6. Due to transient reduction in bilirubin conjugation in liver; therefore hyperbilirubinemia is unconjugated (indirect). Usually requires no treatment.
18. ABO/Rh incompatibility: On day 1. Rh negative mother with Rh positive foetus and may cause hydrops fetalis (generalized edema, including pulmonary edema, with high output heart failure). Treatment is exchange transfusion or plasmapheresis.
19. Sepsis-related: Treat with antibiotics and use phototherapy.
20. Breast-milk jaundice: On day 4-7. Long chain fatty acids in breast milk competitively inhibit glucuronyl transferase activity. Treatment is to substitute formula feed for 2-4 days, then resume breast milk.
21. Others: GI obstruction in foetus (increases enterohepatic circulation), hereditary spherocytosis, drug-induced, breakdown of cephalohematoma, hypothyroidism.
22. Conjugated hyperbilirubinemia in TORCH infections, metabolic disorders, sepsis, obstructive jaundice, and neonatal hepatiis.

Cases 1: Physiological jaundice Case 2: Breast milk jaundice.

Vomiting

Case1: Baby 8 months age is vomiting for the last four months. H/o vomits after feed, while in color, normal weight gain
Case2: Baby 5 months age is vomiting for the last 12 hours. No fever. H/o Job loss, Financial problems, Yellow card (growth chart) shows head circumference 55 cm

1. Confirm the age, first baby? Sex? Siblings?
2. Ask when exactly did it start? Since the first day of life? Ask about choking,
3. Coughing, drooling, cyanosis when feeding, respiratory distress? Real vomiting? Spitting up milk? Gurgling
4. Analyze vomiting: frequency, volume, color (bilious v/s non-bilious), consistency, relation to sucking (during, after), how long after, projectile, can the baby keep anything down?
5. Associated symptoms: Weight loss, pain, jaundice, appetite (hungry baby?), playful? Diarrhea, cough, SOB, wheezing, strider, excessive crying? diuresis? Soiling diaper? LOC, dehydration, rashes, abdominal distention, teething.
6. Feeding H/o: Change in diet, new formula, and breastfeeding, supplements newly introduced? Overfeeding?
7. Birth H/o: Infections, term delivery, problems bee/after, polyhydramnios, meconium, malmations, VATER.
8. PMH.
9. Medications, allergies, vaccinations.
10. Family H/o: Congenital diseases, similar problems in siblings.
11. Impact in growth and development: Weight loss?
12. Thank the mother and address her questions.
13. Start treating this patient with NS 20 ml/kg bolus, then calculate maintenance.
14. Order abdominal USG.

Cases:
1. Normal 2. Child abuse

Case3: A mother with her 6 wk old who has been vomiting for 3 days. Take H/o. Investigations show a palpable mass in the right epigastrium, metabolic hypochloremic alkalosis, and a positive esophageal string sign on barium swallow. What is the diagnosis? Give a DDx for vomiting in an infant.

H/o of infant vomiting: onset, chronology, association with feeling or body position, description of force, volume, colour, composition (bilious, fecal, blood), getting worse or better, is child still hungry afterward or does he settle.

Coughing or gagging with feeds (tracheoesophageal fistula).

Associated diarrhea, constipation, fever, weight loss, abdominal distension, urination. Are other children sick? Has child been in contact with an infected person?

Pregnancy and birth H/o. Development H/o: age and weight normograms.

Feeding H/o: Quantity, frequency, breast v/s formula (which?), feeding difficulties.

PMH, medications, family H/o, ROS.

Diagnosis: Pyloric stenosis

DDx or infant vomiting: congenital malformation (pyloric stenosis, tracheoesophageal fistula, duodenal atresia), gastroenteritis, overfeeding, reflux, food allergy, milk protein intolerance, systemic infection.

Diarrhea

Case1: Mrs. X brings her 6 month old son with diarrhea for 2 days. Take H/o.
Case2: Mrs. X brings 9 month old son with a 3 week H/o of diarrhea. Take H/o.

1. OCD: Establish the timing (> or < than 2 weeks). Is it getting worse?
2. Analyze the diarrhea: How many times/day, every diaper?
3. Amount, color, odor, blood/mucus/pus, nights as well (irritable bowel syndrome does not have diarrhea at night; whereas inflammatory bowel disease has).
4. Character of urine, changes in neurological status.
5. Associated symptoms: Fever, vomiting, URTI (runny nose, cough, wheezing, ear pulling—viral URTI are followed by diarrhea; cough with runny nose followed by diarrhea is typical).
6. Abdominal pain, flatulence, colic, rashes, teething, appetite, weight loss, drop in percentiles (head circumference, height), hungry baby/playful/happy? pallor, dehydration (diuresis, lethargic, crying without tears, cold hands/feet), seizures.
7. Feeding H/o: Breast fed, formula fed, cow's milk, new food introduced?
8. PMH: of relevance: CF, respiratory diseases, allergies, celiac disease, IBD.
9. Medications, immunizations.
10. Birth H/o:
11. Developmental and social H/o: Child neglect, daycare attendance, other kids with diarrhea, siblings, travels.
12. Family H/o:
13. Child neglet must be kept in mind.
14. Management: Make sure that the baby is not in shock. If in shock give normal saline 10 mgm/kg (3 times if needed).
15. If not in shcok check lytes and acid base status. Calculate fluid deficit by the following formula: 100 cc/kg wt/day for the 1st 10 kg wt; 50 cc/kg wt/day for the 2nd 10 kg wt; 20cc/kg wt/day/thereafter. Give the half of the deficit over the first 8 hours and the other half over the next 16 hours.

Cases:
1: Acute gastroenteritis
2: Chronic diarrhea secondary to organic cause

Pallor

Case1: Mrs. X brings 10 month old son because she believes he is pale-Take H/o
Case2: A mother is worried that her 1 yr old looks pale. Take a H/o. Finding: Breast fed for the first 2 months, then 2% milk. What is the most likely diagnosis? What investigations would you order?

1.   OCD: when did she first notice her child pale?
2.   Analyze symptoms of anemia: Sleepy, fatigue, irritable, weak, lethargic, syncope.
3.   Associated symptoms:
     GI bleeding: Melena, hematochezia, diarrhea, pain
     CTD: Rashes, joint pain, eye symptoms, weight loss.
     Infectious diseases: Fever, lymph nodes, rashes, cough.
     GI diseases: Diarrhea, bloating, flatus, GER, anal fissures/prolapse, petechiae, weight loss, steatorrhea.
     Hematological diseases/malignancies: easy bruising, bone pain, fever.
     Lead toxicity.
4.   Precipitating factors: Viral illness, drugs, transfusions, new food.
5.   Feeding H/o: Breastfeeding, iron supplements, formula, cow's milk, solid food, new food lately?
6.   Mother's diet: Calculate the calories needed—[(body weight in pounds x10) + 600] calories
6.   PMH: Of relevance: PUD, GER, CF, CTD, Henoch Shenolein, anaemia.
7.   Medications (sulfas and ABs, NSAIDS), allergies, vaccinations.
8.   Birth H/o:
9.   Developmental and social H/o: Child neglect, abuse.
10.   Family H/o: Hematologic diseases.

Case: Fe deficiency anemia

Chronic Cough

Case 1: Mrs. X brings her 1 year old son with a 6 week H/o of cough. Interview her and address her questions.

1. OCD: Establish the timing (< or > 1 month). Why did you decide to come today? Is it getting worse? Does your son look sick?
2. Analyze the cough: day/night, dry/productive, color, amount, odor, blood. How does the cough sound like: barking = croup; haking = bronchiolitis; whopping = pertusis. Does the cough get worse with change in position? Does he cough more during the night? Sleep well?
3. Precipitating factors: Foreign body, URTI, allergens, pets, smoking at home, drugs, cold air, exercise, heating system, carpets, renovations at home, new food, seasonal pattern.
4. Associated symptoms:
   GI diseases: N/V, diarrhea, weight loss, poor appetite, abdominal distention, rectal prolapsed, steatorrhea, reflux, and hoarseness Respiratory diseases: Runny nose, nasal discharge, adenoids, OM, SOB, cyanosis, wheezing, clubbing, fever, rashes, lymph nodes.
   Cardiac diseases: PND, orthopnea, cyanosis, SOB, clubbing.
5. PMH: OM, pneumonia, lung disease, heart disease, GI disease, CF.
6. Medications, allergies, vaccinations.
7. Feeding H/o.
8. Birth H/o: Jaundice, meconium, infections, and respiratory diseases.
9. Developmental and social H/o. Daycare attendance, travels (TB, parasites), siblings with cough.
10. Family H/o: Asthma, eczemas, allergies.
11. Tell that you'd like to examine the child.

Case: Asthma

Case 2: 2 yr old child with 9 wk H/o of cough, on Amoxil for 2 wks. Take H/o. Give a DDx. What investigations would you order?

Prodromal illness, fever, malaise, rhinnorhea, sore throat, SOB, wheeze.
Is cough productive? Any chest pain? Aggravating and relieving factors.
Onset of cough, chronology, time of day (night), worse with exposure to cold air, dust, smoke, exercise, in grassy areas, weedy areas, forests, certain rooms, in bed.
Did symptoms improve with Amoxil?
Allergic symptoms: red eyes, itching, itch in back of throat.

Pets/air conditioning/type of bed linens and pillows (feather, synthetic, foam).
Changes in the child's environment: different bed linens, new room, change of season. Are there smokers in the house?
D/d: Asthma, bronchitis, URTI, chronic sinusitis, rhinitis, TB, recurrent pneumonia, collapsed lung, cystic fibrosis.
Investigations: CXR, CBC, lytes, INR/PTT, urea, creatinine, PFTs (>4 yrs old), sweat chloride test.

Abdominal pain

Case: Mrs. X brings her 10 year old daughter because of abdominal pain. Interview the mother and address her concerns.

1. OCD
2. Is it recurrent? How many attacks in the last 3 months? (>3 attacks in the last 3 months = Recurrent abdominal pain (RAP).
3. Analyze the pain: PQRST, relationship with meals, stress, situations (school, exams), does it awake the child from sleep? Is the child free of pain on weekends, vacation? Ask about school phobia.
4. Associated symptoms: Fever, N/V, diarrhea, constipation, poor appetite, weight loss, headaches, leg pain (growing pain), dysuria, hematuria, vaginal discharge, periods.
5. PMH: PUD, IBD, sickle cell disease, heart diseases, psychiatric disorders, hospitalizations, surgeries, traumas.
6. Medications, allergies, immunizations.
7. Birth/developmental: R/o child abuse. Ask about pubertal development.
8. HEEADSS questions: emphasize schooling, teacher's reports, family problems, child personality.
9. Red flags: Recurrent abdominal pain: weight loss, fever, joint pain, rash, bleeding, pain away from umbilicus, awake from sleep, diarrhea, vomiting, incontinence, poor appetite.
10. Family H/o: Recurrent abdominal pain, migraine, malignancies.

Case: RAP

Failure to thrive and neglect

Case 1: Mrs. Y brings her 2 year old son because she thinks that he is not growing properly. Interview her.

Case 2: Mrs. S brings her 3 year old daughter to your office because she does not speak as her peers. Take the H/o and address Mrs. S's questions.

Case 3: Mr. K brings his 3 year old son to ER because of an injury in the right arm. The X-rays show spiral # of the right humerus. While the child is treated, you are asked to talk to the father. Interview him.

Case 4: Mrs. X came to your office to see you. She is concerned about her 15 month-old son who is not walking yet. Interview her and take a full developmental H/o.

Case 5: Mrs. D comes to see you because she is concerned about her son being shorter than his peers. Take the H/o and discuss her concerns.

Case 1
1.   OCD: when was first noticed? (Growth chart alteration?) Who noticed? Were serial measurements done? Ask for weight/height/head circumference.
2.   Analyze the main symptom: Weight loss: birth weight, maximum weight, current weight, onset, course and duration of weight loss. Ask about general well being, energy level, activity, symptoms and complaints.
3.   PMH: review the systems: Respiratory, cardiac, GI, infections, kidney, MSK, neurologic, congenital diseases. Review office visits according to his age, hospitalizations, accidents, trauma, and surgeries.
4.   Feeding H/o: What exactly does the child eat = give an example? amount? frequency? How many times per day? Where does the child eat = in the room, kitchen, in front of the TV, distraction?
5.   Who is present during the feeding sessions (mother, father, child alone, entire family, nanny?), When does the child eat? Set times? How parents facilitate feeding? Behavior during feeding—picky eater?
6.   Choking, cyanosis, regurgitation, appears hungry?
7.   Birth H/o: Antenatal H/o—alcohol, smoking, drugs, natal/postnatal complications.
8.   Developmental H/o: brief milestone assessment, age.
9.   Social H/o: Support at home, stressors, attitude toward the child (difficult child?), Who take care of him? daycare, nanny, neighbors.
10. Financial status, state of family.
11. Risk factors for child abuse.
12. Medications, allergies, immunization.

13. Family H/o: Diseases running in the family, parents' and sibling's weight/height.

Note: FTT is a sign or symptom and NOT a disease.

Case 2

1. When was first noticed? Was the child speaking bee? And then stopped speaking?

2. Analyze the speech: Is English the first language spoken at home? How many words, sentences does the child use according to her age? Does she seem to understand when you talk to her? Obey? Respond to noises? Does she use gestures to supplement her limited verbal expression? How does she express herself? Does she stop speaking in selected situations? Echolalia? Sing-song speech? Can she speak to her peers, parents, siblings, and strangers?

   Any teacher's report? Is she a not-listening child?

3. Associated symptoms:

   Hearing problems: H/o of recurrent OM. Ask about detailed audiograms.

   MR: Down's syndrome features, other diseases.

   Maturation delays: Late bloomers in the family.

   Autism: Irritability, routine activities, and social withdrawal.

   CP: Lethargy, abnormal movements, ataxia, spasticity, seizures.

   Psychosocial deprivation: Child stimulation at home, delay in other areas of milestones.

   Other conditions: visual problems, infections, diarrhea, cough, headache, weight loss, short stature.

4. PMH: Prenatal/natal/postnatal: Meningitis, seizures, CP, jaundice, anoxia, hemorrhagia, trauma in the head, infections (TORCHES), OM.

5. Medications, allergies, immunizations

6. Developmental H/o in detail: Gross motor, fine motor, social and language. Concern if red flags are present.

7. Social H/o: Does she play with others?, shy, friendly, eye contact, stereotypical body movements, gesture, dyslexia, compulsive behavior, toilet training, over-dependent with parents.

8. Family situation: Child neglect, siblings, nutrition, stress, family conflicts/situation/finances.

9. Family H/o: Diseases running in the family, anybody with similar problems?

Case 3

1. This is a difficult station where the parent may confront you. So be ready for that. Be gentle but firm. A spiral # of the humerus is highly suspicious of physical child abuse.

2. Start reassuring that the child is been treated the # and is going to be fine. Start asking about the episode: OCD: when did it happen, time lag, if several hrs bee, why did the parent bring the child now? Who was at home? When did that happen? Where were you? Did you see it? Describe the sequence of events. Did the child loss consciousness? Cried? Moved the limb after? How was at night? Other kids at home? "I know that you want the best for your child"

3. Risk factors child abuse.
    Child: Premature, sick, unplanned pregnancy, difficult child, hyperactive, youngest, disappointed with his/her sex, frequent visits to Dr's office, diarrhea, URTI.
    Parents: Unemployed, single, jealous boyfriend/girlfriend, stepfather, parents themselves were victims of abuse, alcohol, drug abuse, medical/psychiatry diseases, problems with the law.
    Parent-child relationship: Stress at home, who feeds the child/takes care of, how much time the parents spend with the kid, how do the parents punish the kid. What is your expectation from your child?
    Social: Isolated family, marital status, financial problems, domestic violence, poverty, incomplete immunizations, and unexplained absences in the school.

4. PMH: Diseases of relevance in prenatal/natal/postnatal period, ER visits, hospitalizations, FD' office visits, fractures, injuries, accidents, traumas, surgeries.

5. Developmental H/o: In detail to find out if delay in milestones.

6. Feeding H/o:

7. Medications/allergies.

8. Keep it cool, address the parent questions and gently say: "The H/o you just gave me about your son/daughter injury is not enough to explain such an important injury".

9. Say that you are concerned about the child and you'd like to hospitalize the child.
    I suspect child abuse/neglect and 1 am going to report it to the CAS.
    I want to help you and I can put you in contact with a social worker.
    The parent may get upset...start screaming, swearing...keep it cool.....
    10. If the parent wants to take their child, tell them that they cannot do it. You can keep the patient in hospital in Canada.

Case 4

1. Start asking the mother why did she decide to come today? Then OCD about the main issue: since when have you noticed that your son did not walk? Did he walk bee?
2. Analyze the gait according to his age: is he able to roll over, sit up, creep, crawl, and stand up by pulling? Cruising? Does he favor one side of his body? = handedness that develops bee 1 year may indicate spastic hemiplegia.
3. Take a full developmental H/o: Go through the milestones: Always give examples.
   Gross motor skills: How old was he when able to: hold up the head, head control, roll over, sit, creep, crawl, pull to stand, cruise?
   Fine motor skills: At what age was he able to: fist, unfist, reach and grab, transfer, rake from surface, immature/mature pincer, voluntary release.
   Language skills: When was he able to smile socially, cooing, orienting to voice, babbling, "mama dada", indiscriminate, gesturing, 1,2,3 words?
   Social skills: Smiles, plays, stranger anxiety.
4. Associated symptoms: Review of systems.
   CP: Abnormal postures, movements, asymmetries, seizures, abnormal posture, tone.
   MR: Other milestones abnormal, Down's syndrome features, other genetic disorders
   Neglect: home situation, other skills affected, siblings, weight/height dropping from chart.
   Other conditions: Physical abnormalities, SOB, cyanosis, lethargic, poor feeding, diarrhea.
5. Feeding H/o: In detail.
6. Birth H/o: Antenatal/natal/postnatal diseases: TORCHES, alcohol, smoking, drugs, IUGR, complications during delivery (fetal distress, trauma, anoxia, jaundice, respiratory distress, infections, and seizures).
7. Medications, allergies, immunizations.
8. Social H/o: Family/home situation: child neglect/abuse.
9. Family H/o: Similar problems or diseases.

Case 5

1. When did you first notice the short stature first noticed? Growth charts? Rate of growth > 5-6 cm/year.
2. How many times the height was measured? Is the weight a concern?
3. Associated symptoms:
   Brain tumors: Headaches, visual problems, hearing problems.

Systemic diseases: bone-joint pain, energy level, poor appetite, weight loss. Constitutional: normal child's heath.

4. PMH: celiac disease, IBD, thyroid, heart, lung, kidney, CF, DM, HTN, endocrinopathies, Sx, hospitalizations, traumas.
5. Medications (steroids), allergies, immunizations.
6. Diet H/o: In detail
7. Birth H/o: Prenatal/natal/postnatal conditions and complications.
8. Developmental H/o: Brief review, schooling, mental status, sports.
9. Signs of puberty: Onset, stage, delayed/precocious.
10. Family H/o: Parental height and age of puberty; growth spurt in the family.
11. Address the parent's concerns.

Case 1: FTT secondary to child neglect
Case 2: Speech delay secondary to recurrent OM
Case 3: Child abuse
Case 4: Motor skill delay secondary to CP
Case 5: Constitutional short stature

Enuresis

Case: Mrs. X brings her 7 year old son because he has been wetting the bed lately. Interview her and address her questions.

1. Perceive the severity of the problem in the family and show concern. Confirm the age of the child, ask why she come now? Is it just enuresis or also encopresis?
2. Analyze the episode: Was the child continent ever? How many times a week happen? Is it occurring at night/day or both? What did she try to do so far? Any investigations done? Relation to activity, is it getting more often?
3. Associated symptoms: review the systems:
   UTI: Dysuria, urinary frequency, urgency, weight loss, fever, abdominal pain.
   DM: Polydipsia, polyuria, weight loss
   Neurological causes: Seizures, headaches, and visual problems
   Diabetes insipius: Headaches, visual problems, limping
   Respiratory conditions: Adenoids, tonsil hypertrophy
   Sleep disorders: Night terrors, nightmares
   MR: School marks, developmental delay.
4. Find stressors: Recent move, birth of a sibling, death of a loved one, school phobia, peer problems, family situation, neglect/abuse, divorce.
5. PMH: Prenatal/natal/postnatal diseases. Particularly R/o: neurogenic bladder, spinal cord abnormalities, UTI, DM, DI.
6. Medications, allergies, immunizations
7. Developmental and social H/o.
8. Risk factors for enuresis: kidney diseases, family H/o of enuresis.
9. Management: Urine analysis for glucose, protein, WBCs, specific gravity, urine culture, counseling, buzzer and alarm system that operates when the bed sheet become wet. Tricyclic antidepressants.

Hyperactive child

Case: Mrs. X brings her 7 year old son because his teacher advised an assessment for ADD. Interview the mother.

1.   Do you have any letter from the teacher? Same school? Same teacher? What did the teacher tell you exactly?
2.   OCD: when did you first notice this behavior (>6m)? How old was he? Have you seen anybody other than me (psychiatrist.), give me a specific example of his behavior…What make it worse/better?
3.   Investigate the 3 areas:

Diagnosis: Persistent pattern, before age 7 at least in 2 settings (home and school)

a. Inattention:
Fails to pay attention/careless mistakes
Unable to sustain attention
Does not seem to listen
Difficulty organizing tasks
Easily distracted
Often forgetful in daily activities
Avoids tasks that require sustained mental effort
Fail to finish chores, homework?
Does he loose things e.g. pencils, books?
Does external stimulus easily distract him?

b. Hyperactivity:
Does he have problems sitting still?
Fidgets with hands/feet?
Leaves the seat in classroom when not suppose to?
Acts as if driven by a motor?
Difficulty waiting for his turn?
Fidgets hands and feet
Runs about or climbs excessively the situation
Talks excessively
Blurts
Interrupts or intrudes on others

c. Impulsivity:
Does he answer before finishing the questions?

Interrupts others? Brake the rules?
Bits other kids, steal things?

4.   Associated symptoms:
      Neurological diseases: Headaches, seizures, vision loss
      Ear problems: Hearing loss, OM, psychiatric diseases, school phobia, anxiety. Depression, bipolar, defiant, tics
      Organic diseases: Abdominal pain, weight loss, enuresis, and encopresis
      Sleep disorders: Night-terrors/nightmares.
      MR: Head-banging, delay in different areas and skills.
5.   PMH: antenatal/natal/postnatal H/o: Complications (meningitis, seizures, anoxia, jaundice), planned pregnancy, weight/height, term-preterm, medications, alcohol, drugs, and smoking. HTN, DM, trauma, accidents, hospitalizations, surgeries.
6.   Developmental H/o: Milestone in detail diet: breakfast bee going to school?
7.   Medications, allergies, immunizations.
8.   School performance: Assess reading comprehension, spelling, writing problems, composition, calculation, solving process.
9.   Social H/o: Family group, siblings, friends, divorce, loss of a loved one, domestic/child abuse, substance abuse, financial stress, single parent, chronic diseases, inappropriate expectations, chaotic home environment, attachment disorders.
10.   Family H/o: ADD in the family, psychiatric disorders.

Fever

Case 1: Mrs. X brought her 13 months old son because he presented with fever since yesterday and 1 hour ago had a "fit". She is terrified. Take the H/o and try to find out what happened.
Case 2: You are going to talk to Mrs. X, mother of a 9 month old baby. Mrs. X tells you that her baby has fever since 2 days. Interview her and her questions.
Case 3: Mrs. X brings her 3 week old baby to ER because she noticed that the baby was "cranky" and feverish. Take a full H/o and address her concerns.

Case1:
1.   Show concern about the mother being distressed. Reassure. Ask where the baby is? Who is taking care of the baby now? Is he awake? Alert? Playing? Then start asking about the episode. Remember that you are going to take the H/o from the mother.
2.   Onset: what do you mean by "FITS"? Describe the episode:
     Before: what was the baby doing? How did it happen? Where did it happen? Witnesses…
     During: LOC? How long? Was he stiff, tights up, shaking? Drooling, cyanosis, vomiting? Eyes rolling? Did he hit the head?
     After: drowsiness, Todd's paralysis, how quickly regained consciousness? Confusion, cranky, alert, crying, limb movements? Did he look in pain? What did you do?
3.   Analyze the fever: Height, pattern, and duration (how fast the temperature went up?)
     Did you check the temperature? How? Medications?
4.   Try to find out etiology:
     Prior febrile seizures?
     URTI: Runny nose, cough, SOB, wheezing, cyanosis, pulling ears
     Meningitis: Lethargy, focal seizures, floppy, rejected food, less playful, poor sucking.
     Eruptive diseases: Skin rashes in detail
     GE: N/V, diarrhea
     Head trauma, toxins (lead)
5.   PMH: Birth H/o (prenatal/natal/postnatal diseases or complications)
6.   Immunizations: Up to date? Any vaccines recently?
7.   Medications; allergies.
8.   Feeding H/o: Gaining weight? Type of feed.
9.   Brief developmental H/o: Ask according to age, include social H/o
10. Criteria for benign febrile seizure:

Febrile (>38° C; usually associated with rapid increase of temperature)

Age: 6 months to 5 years

Not focal (generalized)

Neurologically fine (no focal seizure)

Lasts less than 15 minutes and no recurrence within 24 hours

Family H/o

11. Risk factor the first F. Seizure: Family H/o, neonatal discharge from hospital after 28 days, developmental delay, child care attendance, very high temperature, low sodium.

12. When you finish reassure the parents and think: a) Do you have to admit the patient? b) In which cases do you hospitalized? c) Risk of recurrence? d) Explain to the parents the condition e) Management.

Seizure

Case1: 2 yr old child with H/o of fever and 1 seizure. Counsel the parents.

1. A typical febrile seizure is a brief, generalized tonic-clonic seizure related to high fever (at least 39ºC) and occurring between the ages of 3 months and 7 yrs.
2. The post-seizure stage is characterized by improvement in confusion and lethargy.
3. The greatest risk factor for febrile seizures is an H/o of febrile seizures in the parents.
4. Seizures may be the result of fever from any cause, including post-immunization.
5. In the absence of an abnormal developmental H/o (CP, developmental delay), they are usually benign.
6. Seizures do not cause mental impairment unless they are prolonged (> 30 min); but can be a symptom of brain damage.
7. Prognosis after a single febrile seizure: 65% will never have another seizure, 30% will have further febrile seizures, 3% will go on to have seizures without fever, and 2% will develop lifelong epilepsy.
8. Treatment: Control fever with acetaminophen (Tylenol) and use sublingual ativan 1 mg po/sl/pr if a seizure occurs at home. Turn patient onto the side, do not force objects or fingers into mouth.
9. Bring to ER if seizure does not stop within 10 min.
10. Patient should be investigated with CT head and EEG. Prophylactic anticonvulsant therapy is a consideration with repeated seizures.

Case2: 16 yr old male with 3 episodes of sudden loss of awareness lasting <1 minute, wants information on epilepsy. Counsel.

1. Cause of seizures: Disturbed electrical activity in the brain, often with a tiny focus of abnormal tissue from previous infection, trauma including birth trauma or inherited.
2. Absence or petit-mal seizure starts in young people. 1/3 of cases resolve spontaneously with age.
3. Seizures do not damage the brain unless they are prolonged (>30 min) and absence seizures are not associated with decreased intelligence or learning ability.
4. Most people with this type of epilepsy are well controlled on medication and have no limitations in their activities, careers or relationships.

5. The 2 main treatment issues are choosing the right medications to achieve seizure control without excessive sedation and avoiding dangerous activities such as driving, mountain climbing, swimming alone, operating machinery, until good control is achieved.

6. You must not drive at present. The MOT requires a full year seizure-free activity before they will grant or renew a driver's license to people with epilepsy.

7. Inform patient that you will notify the MOT and that you are required by law to do so.

8. Sleep deprivation, alcohol, and many medications lower seizure threshold, so the patient should be careful to obtain adequate rest, should not drink at all, and should consult a physician before taking other medications.

9. Outline a treatment plan consisting of investigations: EEG, CT head, metabolic screen, mediations (drugs of choice for absence: ethosuximide and valproate), follow-up appointments.

10. Get parents involved.

Meningitis

1. Name, age, onset of symptoms, duration, increasing or decreasing in severity, fever, nausea, vomiting, photophobia, phonophobia, neck stiffness, headache, rash.
2. Medications or other interventions tried?
3. H/o of severity, chronology of migraine, premonitory visual disturbance? Recent neurosurgery? Head trauma?
4. Other illness? Contacts with meningitis at school or work?
5. Medications, drugs, alcohol, allergies, PMH, family H/o, ROS.
6. P/E: Vitals, GCS, note general appearance of patient, if patient is very ill, orientation.
7. Inspect for meningococcemial rash.
8. Cranial nerves: Pupillary reflexes, note photophobia if present, extraocular muscle movement, check for double-vision, visual fields, facial sensation and movement, gross hearing, sternocleidomastoid and trapezius power.
9. Tone: Passive rapid movement at elbows, rotation of forearms, flexion/extension of knees.
10. Cerebellar testing: Finger-nose, heel-shin, rapid alternating movements or forearms.
11. Power at deltoids, triceps, biceps, wrist extension and flexion, finger abduction and adduction, psoas, quadriceps, hamstrings, ankle dorsiflexion and plantar flexion.
12. Deep tendon reflexes at triceps, biceps, brachioradialis, knee, ankle, Babinski.
13. Light touch, pinprick over limbs and body, vibration sense at joints.
14. Signs of meningismus: Kernig's sign—pain in the neck on extension of the knee with the hip in 90° of flexion. Brudzinski's sign—pain on passive flexion of the neck.
15. Investigations: CBC, lytes, INR/PTT, BUN, Cr, blood cultures, ABG, CT head followed by lumbar puncture if H/o and P/E are suspicious for raised ICP (lumbar puncture may, rarely, precipitate brain herniation in the presence of raised ICP).
16. Treatment: Initiate IV antibiotics immediately (before head CT and LP) if the clinical picture is suspicious for meningitis. Cefuroxime 2 g IV q 4hr + ampicillin 50 mg/kg IV q 6 hr. Consult ICU. Consider intubation and intensive management of ICP.

Child abuse

Case1: 22 month old female child brought to ER by her mother with fractured left humerus. Two previous fractures in past 3 months, bruises seen on forehead. Manage. Case2: Child with vomiting and crying. Once you take the H/o, it turns out that it is normal vomiting or non-specific crying.

1. Warning signs of child abuse.
2. Risk factors for child abuse: Social isolation, poverty, substance abuse, jealousy between boyfriend and father, parent's abused themselves, personality/character disorder or mental illness, difficult child.
3. H/o: How did the injury happen? Who was looking after the child when it happened? Who are the child's caregivers and who lives in the house or comes in contact with the child? How did the child get the bruises? What happened with the other fractures?
4. Any other injuries in the past? Is the child accident prone or difficult to handle?
5. What is the child's personality: open v/s withdrawn.
6. Are there other children in the house?
7. Have they had broken bones or other injuries?
8. Was this child a planned pregnancy, problems with pregnancy, birth H/o.
9. Milestones: Where does the child live (isolation), income level of parents, problems with the law, alcoholism, drug use, smoking by caregivers or other adults in the home?
10. What is the typical response of caregivers when the child cries or misbehaves?
11. Were the caregivers abused as children?
12. Is there spousal abuse, sexual abuse, sexual abuse or incest?
13. Has the Children's aid society been involved with this child or other children? Interview relatives, friends.
14. Child's medical H/o, medications, allergies.
15. P/E: observe child's behaviour.
16. Inspect for malnutrition, bruises, scars, burns especially on the flexor surfaces.
17. Inspect oral cavity, perineum, anus, genitalia. Ophthalmoscope for retinal hemorrhages (shaken baby syndrome).
18. Evaluate for development. Neurological exam for possible brain injury.
19. Investigations: X-rays for old fractures if records not available. CBC, lytes, urea, Cr, INR/PTT, albumin (malnutrition).

20. Explanation doesn't match the injury, delay in seeking treatment, recent family crisis, unrealistic expectations of child behaviour by caregivers.
21. Treatment: Admit for child's safety and investigations; consult child psychiatrist and pediatric orthopedic surgeon.
22. Physicians have to report suspicion of child abuse to CAS.
23. Family therapy, frequent follow-up to monitor development.

Dysuria

1. Investigations: midstream clean catch voided urine specimen.
2. May need to catheterize or aspirate suprapubically to obtain a good specimen.
3. Urine dipstick, microscopy, culture and sensitivity.
4. If child appears systemically ill, take blood for cultures, CBC, Urea, Cr, lytes.
    Renal U/S for major malformations and voiding cysto-urethrogram (VCUG) should be done in all children 6 yrs old or less with UTI.
5. Radiological investigations may be postponed until the second UTI in girls over 6 yrs old due to higher rate of benign UTI.
6. Postpone the VCUG 3-6 wks to allow normalization of flow after UTI.
7. Counselling: Ask why the mother is concerned about sexual abuse? UTI alone is not a good indicator. Explain that, in girls, UTIs are common because of short urethra and proximity to anal area.
8. Describe front to back wiping after urination, and general hygiene.
9. Give prescription for Septran 8-12 mg/kg/day PO BD x 7-10 days if urine dipstick positive for white cells and patient not allergic to Septran.
10. Arrange follow-up in 2 weeks for re-culture of urine. Explain need for U/S and VCUG to rule out flow abnormalities which may threaten kidney function, arrange these.
11. Consider hospitalization for pyelonephritis or rehydration.

Asthma

Case: 4 yr old boy with cough for 6 wks. No improvement on antibiotics 3 weeks ago. Take H/o. What is your DDx? Give the most likely diagnosis and describe a treatment plan.

1. H/o: Prodromal illness, fever, malaise, rhinorhea, sore throat, SOB, wheeze.
2. Is the cough productive? Any chest pain?
3. Aggravating and relieving factors, onset of cough, chronology, time of day (night), worse with exposure to cold air, dust, smoke, exercise, in grassy areas, weedy areas, forests, certain rooms, in bed.
4. Allergic symptoms: Red eyes, itching, itch in back of throat.
5. Family pets, air conditioning, type of bed clothes and pillows (feather, synthetic, foam), Recent change in the child's environment: new room, change of season?
6. Are there smokers in the house? PMH, medications, allergies, family H/o of asthma?
7. DDx: Asthma, bronchitis, URTI, chronic rhinitis, sinusitis, TB, recurrent pneumonia, collapsed lung, CF.
8. Most likely Dx: Asthma.
9. Treatment: Steroids are the key treatment. Oral steroids can be given in a short course if inhaled steroids are ineffective.
10. Ventolin (albuterol) can be used on a prn (when necessary) basis.
11. Modify the home environment to decrease contact with common allergens: dust mites, pollen, pet hair.
12. Control dust with thorough and regular cleaning.
13. Boil bed clothes, plastic undercovers on mattress and pillows, remove rugs, install air conditioner, remove pets, no smoking in the house (second-hand smoke is a cause of childhood asthma).
14. Warn parents of the symptoms of a severe asthma attack (status asthmaticus) and when to come to the ER.
15. Discuss treatment strategy: A regular anti-immune medication i.e. steroid or sodium cromoglycate, with prn bronchodilator.
16. H/o: Symptoms of hypercalcemia: fatigue, muscle weakness, arthralgias, renal colic due to nephrolithiasis, emotional lability (can progress to psychosis and coma), bone pain, abdominal pain, nausea, vomiting, constipation, ileus, polyuria, polydypsia, nocturia.
17. Onset and duration of these.
18. Malignancy symptoms: Weight loss, night sweats, fatigue.
19. Orthostatic hypotension (Addison's).

20. Heat intolerance, hyperactivity (hyperthyroidism).
21. Diet especially amount of milk, use of calcium supplements and antacids.
22. Medications, drugs and alcohol, smoking, allergies, PMH (heartburn, reflux, gastritis, peptic ulcer), family H/o (multiple endocrine neoplasia—MEN).
23. ROS.
24. P/E: Trousseau's sign (inflate BP cuff, leave on 1-2 min, distal arm goes into tetanic flexion, indicates hypercalcemia).
25. Inspect for signs of Addison's disease—bronze skin tone, orthostatic hypotension. Cushing's—moon facies, striae, buffalo hump.
26. Chest: palpate sternum and ribs for bone pain.
27. Examine breasts for signs of malignancy dimpling, masses.
28. General cardiopulmonary exam.
29. Abdominal exam: Palpate liver carefully for masses, percuss kidneys for pain.
30. Rectal: test stool for occult blood.
31. Examine long bones for straightness and tenderness—Paget's disease of bone.
32. DDx: Parathyroid adenoma (hyperparathyroidism) due to inherited MEN (also have pituitary adenoma causing Addison's or Cushing's), malignancy (myeloma, lung, breast, squamous in any site), Paget's disease of bone, hyperthyroidism, vitamin D in pharmacologic doses, milk-alkali syndrome (large ingestion of milk and alkali, usually gastric hyperacidity).
33. Investigations: CBC, lytes, Bun, Cr, albumin, AST, ALT, Alkaline phosphatase, GGT, INR/PTT, serum cortisol, serum PTH, ionized serum calcium, serum phosphate, TSH, serum protein electrophoresis (for monoclonal gammopathy of myeloma).
34. Plain X-rays of tender or malformed bones, including skull (see salt and pepper lesions).
35. CT head, thyroid, adrenals.

Child not speaking

1. H/o of not speaking should determine whether the problem is primary (never spoke) or secondary (stopped speaking).
2. Secondary causes of mutism are psychological upset (due to family discord, etc.) and rare inherited neurodegenerative conditions.
3. Primary mutism may be part of a global developmental delay or related to hearing problems which are either congenital (inherited, intrauterine infections—rubella, CMV, toxoplasmosis) or acquired (postnatal sepsis, meningitis, recurrent ear infections, ototoxic drugs esp. streptomycin, trauma).
4. Pregnancy and birth H/o: Mother ill while pregnant? Rubella, CMV, toxoplasmosis, perinatal or later infections (meningitis).
5. Medications given in the past, family H/o of deafness or late speaking.
6. Developmental H/o (from parent): Growth—expected height and weight for age?
7. Speech—Has child ever spoken words or phrases, are these used appropriately?
8. Has the child made sounds? Chronology and description of these.
9. How does the child communicate if not through speech?
10. Gross motor—When did child start walking, running?
11. Fine motor—When did you notice pincer grasp, turning pages in a book.
12. Selected developmental milestones:

Speech	6 months	imitates sounds, eye contact
	12 months	2 words beyond mama and dada
	24 months	2-3 word phrases
	2-3 yrs	short sentences
Gross motor	6 months	roll over
	9 months	stand
	12 months	cruise
	15 months	walk
Fine motor	12 months	pincer grasp
	24 months	turns pages in a book
Social	6 months	stranger anxiety
	9 months	separation anxiety
	2 yrs	says "no"
	5 yrs	writes name

13. Hearing: Does the child wake up in response to sounds? Startle to loud sounds?

14. Comes when called? Understand spoken instructions?
15. H/o of ear infections, wax problems? Ask about swimming.
16. PMH, medications, allergies, family H/o, ROS.
17. Diagnosis: Given recurrent otitis media with poor hearing the most likely diagnosis is retarded speech development due to poor hearing.
18. Refer to ENT for hearing tests, tympanic drainage etc.

Immunization

Case: Young mother with 6 wk old baby has recently emigrated from Ghana. Poor English skills. Concerned about whether she should have her baby immunized. Counsel.

Be aware of the communication barriers such as language difficulties to understand the patient's objectives, fears, preconceptions to deal with these in an empathetic non-judgmental way to transmit information in a way that is consistent with the patient's expectations and understandable to them, and to invite further questions and feedback.

1. Ask if the patient would prefer someone perhaps a family member to translate.
2. Ask about the patient's concerns, what does she want to know and why?
3. Vaccines protect children from diphtheria, tetanus, pertussis, polio (DPTP) mumps, rubella, measles (MMR), influenza (Hib) and hepatitis (HepB).
4. These diseases were once common and caused serious, sometimes fatal illnesses and all of which are now hardly ever seen because of vaccines.
5. Because the vaccines stimulate the immune system, some children have a temporary sore arm at the site of injection, malaise, mild fever, or rash. It is very rare to have a more serious reaction (seizures, encephalopathy have been reported).
6. Standard modern vaccines are not known to cause disease or to have long term deleterious effects.
7. Compare these risks with the risk of not being vaccinated.
8. Explain the recommended immunization schedule (below) and give the patient some information pamphlets, invite further questions and ask her to return in two weeks for the child's first immunization.
9. Contraindications to vaccination: Previous serious reaction to vaccine. Special contraindications to MMR, which is a live attenuated vaccine suspended in egg white protein and preserved with neomycin: allergy to egg or neomycin, pregnancy, and immunocompromised state.
10. Special contraindications to the pertussis component of DPTP (which is thought to be the component responsible for seizures and encephalopathic reactions when they occur) = progressive neurologic epilepsy.

Recommended immunization schedule:
2 months   DPTP, Hib (Pentavalent vaccine)
4 months   DPTP, Hib (Pentavalent vaccine)

6 months	DPTP, Hib (Pentavalent vaccine)
1 yr.	MMR
18 months	DPTP, Hib (Pentavalent vaccine)
4-6 yr	MMR DPTP
12-13 yr	Hep B (2 vaccinations at an interval of 6 months)
14-16 yr	TdP (certificate of immunization for high school)
Every 10 yr	Td

Alcoholic teenager—counsel

1. Alcohol—impact on family-work-social.
2. 1 drink = beer 12 ounce = wine-5 ounce = hard liquor 1.5 ounce.
3. Low risk is 2 drinks a day or less-high risk is more than that + alcohol related physical or social problems.
4. CAGE—cut down; annoyed at criticism; guilty; eye opener.
5. Complications—alco. cardiomyopathy; Wernicks-peri neuropathy; BP; pancreatitis; liver disease; oesophagus cancer; anxiety, depression; sex dysfunction; fetal damage.
6. Questions: HALT,FATAL,BUMP,DT.
    Drink to get high-drink alone-look forward to drinking-tolerant-family H/o-member AA-tranquilizers-attempt to quit-legal problems-blackouts-used in unplanned way-medicinal reasons-protect ethanol supply-drink and drive-think that you are an alcoholic.
7. Alcoholic anonymous a) OP and day programs—family Rx-Al-Anon-Alteen, screen for spouse and child abuse b) IP programs.
8. Pharmacology—diazepam for withdrawal (Delirium tremens after surgery—Haloperidol—after alcohol-diazepam)—disulfiram—blocks acetaldehyde to acetic acid + reduce BP—Naltrexone-competitive opioid antagonist that reduce cravings.

Section 7

Psychiatry

Eating disorders
Acute delirium
Acute psychosis
Obsessive compulsive disease
Panic attacks
Mania
Depression
Anorexia
Obesity
Mini mental status examination
Hysteria

Eating disorders

Case 1: Ms. X is an 18 year old woman who was brought by her mother to your office because she has lost 20 pounds. Interview her.

Case 2: Ms.X is a 19 year old woman who came with a friend today. Her room mate is worried because Joan has lost 18 pounds lately. Interview her.

1. Why are your mom/friend worry about you?
2. Do you think they are all wrong? Talk to the patient alone.
3. Analyze the weight loss: (>15 % of expected); ask about original weight (bring a picture next time).
4. Has there ever been a time when people gave you a hard time about being too thin or loosing too much weight?
5. What was the lowest you weighed?
6. What is your weight now?
7. Have you tried to lose weight intentionally?
8. What did you do? Have you had binge eating followed by intentional vomiting, laxatives, diuretics, and excessive exercise?
9. Bulimia: have you ever gone on eating binges when you ate abnormally large amounts of food over a short period of time?
10. How much would you eat during a binge?
11. Did you feel you lost control over your eating?
12. To prevent gaining weight, have you force yourself to vomit, go on strict diets, use laxatives, water pills, enemas, exercise vigorously?
13. How many times a week/month?
14. Body image: do you like yourself? How much time a day do you spend thinking about your figure? What happen if you eat, do you feel guilty?
15. Associated symptoms: Have you felt headaches, weakness, dizziness, decrease in energy, cramps, nail braking, dental status, diarrhea, urinary output, palpitations, memory problems, SOB.
16. Psychiatric screening: Mood, depression, anger, suicidal ideation.
17. Diet: Can you describe your daily diet?
18. PMH: Thyroid, DM, asthma, heart, lung, kidney diseases.
19. Medications, allergies.
20. Social H/o: HEEADSS questions (please, see the H/o) in detail, alcohol, smoking, drugs, sexual H/o.
21. LMP: When was your last one?
22. Expectations and ideas about what is going on.
23. Key points: Loss >15% expected weight, lowest weight, body image, dental damage, memory, suicide, explain one day's diet, malignancy, OCD, AIDS.

When you finish the interview, think about:

1. DDX: Bipolar disorder, social phobias, medical conditions (malignancies, AIDS), OCD, body dysmorphic syndrome, bulimia.

2. Do you think you have to admit this patient?

3. Explain what your Dx is, express your concern regarding the meals not being nutritious enough her age and sizes, related-health problems, lack of menses, and risk of osteoporosis. Tell her that a lot of young woman die because of starvation.

4. Develop a plan until the patient reaches the right weight. Stop laxatives, diuretics, supervised meals, weight monitoring.

5. Talk about treatments: Oral intake monitoring, family psychotherapy, treatment of specific psychiatric conditions. Medicaitons: SSRls, Amitriptiline, MAOI.

6. How do you feel about this? Is not going to be easy, but there is a group of people ready to help you. Offer support, long-term F/U, counseling, information.

Acute Delirium

Case 1: A 68 year old man had a hip surgery 48 hrs ago. He is in the surgical ward. The nurse calls you because he can not sleep at night, complaints of loud voices and images coming into the room. Assess him. Do not do a physical.
Case 2: 67 year old woman had a CABG surgery 2 days ago. Today the nurse calls you because she is agitated and wants to leave the hospital. Assess her. Don't do a physical.

Dealing with the station:

1. Delirium is a medical emergency: People can die in the context of delirium (after fall, #, aspiration pneumonia, dehydration, resp. failure, sepsis, lytes disturbance).
2. In this station you may encounter difficulties approaching the patient, so be very gentle since you enter into the room, take your time and do not rush the patient with a lot of questions.
3. Address that the patient looks frightened and ask if you scared him/her. De-escalate the fear.
4. Keep the tract on the patient's speech (hallucinations), and slowly get into the mental exam.
5. Assure that the patient is safe in the hospital.
1. Open questions: I am…..Respect the distance. Ask what is happening?
2. Screening for psychosis: Did you sleep last night? (Hallucinations/delusions) Have you seen/heard/felt…things?
3. Describe them. Invite the patient to sit down if not already sitting.
4. Try to create a safe environment where you are able to communicate with the patient, so the rest is going to be easy.
5. Address how difficult/scared this situation must be for the patient.
6. Ask what she/he wants. Establish that you are a physician and you want to help.
7. Gently start you MMSE: Give time and do not rash.
8. Screening for suicidal ideation.
9. Take a little bit of H/o regarding physical complains: UTI, pneumonia, fever, medications, pain, hypoxemia.
10. Try to find out if the patient was drinking before the Sx. Drug or alcohol withdrawal is always a possibility.
11. Continue reassuring the patient and ask if the patient has any questions. Key points: Do not rush; keep proper distance; invite to sit down, "I understand how difficult it is for you", "I am a doctor".
12. MMSE, capacity assessment and ask for suicidal ideation.

When you finish your station think about:
1. DDx: Delirium v/s Dementia.
2. Are there any treatable precipitating factors that can cause this episode?
3. Outline a safety management (chemical or physical restrain if necessary).
4. Long-term treatment and prognosis.

Acute Psychosis

Case 1: 30 year old man is brought by his wife because he has been acting strange lately.
Case 2: 60 year old woman is complaining of radiation coming from the wall at home.
Case 3: 29 year old man wants you to sign a letter him in which he is complaining of his neighbors who try to get him.
Case 4: A middle aged homeless woman came to ER. The nurse tells you that she did not tell her name and she is acting strangely. Interview her.
Case 5: A young man is brought to ER because of acute agitation and bizarre behavior.

Dealing with the station:
1. This is a station where you may not be able to interact with the patient be ready for it. Just be gentle. Do not approach the patient if she/he looks agitated, keep calm and wait until proper time to ask questions.
2. Your objective is to create a "safe environment" where the patient feels comfortable, secure, and you are able to interact you him/her.
3. Remember that in acute psychosis the patient lacks insight, so she/he may be experiencing disturbing hallucinations. Try to find out what is distressing the patient.
4. You can not leave the room without knowing if this patient is at a high risk of suicide/homicide. In this case, you should certify the patient (i.e. involuntary hospitalization).
5. You should also know if the acute psychosis is secondary to substance abuse.

1. Start asking the patient why she/he is here? Did anybody bring you here? Why?
2. Have the patient been here bee? In another hospital? How many times?
3. Analyze the level of functionality, change in behavior, how long?
4. Precipitating factor: Why now? What happened?
5. If the patient has a chronic psychiatric disease, address compliance to medication.
6. Screening for psychosis: If you see that the patient looks disturbed, distressed, fidgeted, ask: you look frightened to me, what is disturbing you? Probably the voices. So start with the screening.

1) Hallucinations:

Auditory: Can you hear voices that others cannot?

If yes, what did you hear? How many voices?

Are they talking to you or to each other? Are they females/males?

Do you recognize them?

What are they telling you? "To hurt yourself or someone else?" Any commands?

(This gives you an idea of how distressed this patient is and also the risk of suicide/homicide).

Address how difficult this situation must be for the patient.

Visual: Have you ever seen things that no one else can see?

Tactile: Strange sensation in your body or skin? (Something creeping/crawling in your body).

Olfactory: smelling things.

2) Delusions:

Do you think that people are out there to hurt you, anybody is following you?

Do you feel that there is a plot against you e. g: neighbors (Persecutions, paranoid) Have you felt that you are receiving messages from the TV, radio?

Do things look specially arranged for you? (Reference).

Do you think that people can read your thoughts (Thought broadcasting?)

Are your thoughts ever taken out from your head? (Thought withdrawal).

Do you think you have done something terrible and you deserve to be punished? (Delusion of guilt).

Do you think that you are extremely talented and you have a mission to achieve? (Delusion of grandiosity).

Are you concerned about a serious illness that Drs. did not find yet? (Somatic delusion).

Do you do something over and over again even if you know that is unreasonable?

7. Mood screen: Depression (can be schizoaffective disorder). Mania (Bipolar).

8. Suicide/homicide: Have you thought of hurting yourself.

9. In case the patient thinking that there is plot against him/her you may trigger the patient's real thoughts by asking: Do you want to put your neighbors in jail and then what?

10. Screen for anxiety, cognitive, eating disorder.

11. Consciousness, memory, orientation and intelligence are normal in schizophrenia. Verify.

12. Social H/o: Occupation, how are you dealing with your life since you are under a lot of distress?
13. Where do you live? Are you able to take care of yourself? Finances? Employment? Family?
14. Relationship? friends? sex? alcohol, drugs, criminal H/o.
15. PMH and medications + allergies.
16. Family H/o: Psychiatric disorders, substance/domestic abuse.
17. Duration < 1 month—brief psychotic disorder; between 1-6 months—schizophreniform disorder; > 6months—schizophrenia.
18. Identify if also negative symptoms of schizophrenia.

When you finish, think about:
1. DDx according to the timing of the symptoms.
2. Do you have to hospitalize this patient?
3. Explain why: you are under lot of distress, not able to take care of yourself, eat, and sleep.
4. Outline the treatment: psychotherapy and pharmacologic treatment.

Case 1: Brief psychotic disorder; Case 2: Schizophreniform disorder, Case 3: Schizophrenia; Case 4: Schizophrenia; Case 5: Acute psychosis secondary to drugs.

Case: 22 yr old male, hears voices. Take H/o.

H/o with special attention to the chronicity of symptoms, and work, school and relationship histories.

DSM IV criteria for Dx of schizophrenia:
A: 2 or more of the following characteristic symptoms occurring for a significant portion of a 1 month period: Delusion, hallucinations, disorganized speech, catatonic or grossly disorganized behaviour, negative symptoms (flat affect, poverty of speech, anhedonia, affectional impairment).
B: Social or occupational dysfunction.
C: Continuous sign of some disturbance for at least 6 months including severe disturbance in A.
D: Schizoaffective or mood disorder excluded.
E: Substance abuse or general medical condition excluded.
F: If there is a H/o of autistic disorder or pervasive development disorder, then the diagnosis of schizophrenia is made only if delusions or hallucinations are prominent for at least 1 month.

Obsessive compulsive disorder

Case 1: A 30 year old man came to see you. He did not want to explain the reason of his visit. Interview him.
Case 2: A 28 year old woman is brought by her mother because of excessive dryness in the hands. Interview her.

1. Go into the room and greet the patient. If you see that the patient is wearing gloves and does not want to shake hands, do not worry and continue.
2. Start with an open question, what brought you here today? The patient may tell you about being unable to touch things because of contamination with germs, or doing research about bacteria resistance or "super viruses". Take it from there and address the fact that he/she wearing gloves. Ask about level of distress, functioning, and how long has this problem being going on?
3. Start asking about obsessions. Some people are bothered by recurrent thoughts or impulses that seem inappropriate or do not make sense, but they keep repeating over and over again and are difficult to keep it out of their mind. e.g. thoughts about hurting/killing somebody, yelling obscenities in public, inappropriate sexual actions against your moral integrity, being contaminated with germs or dirt.
4. Have you ever experienced one of those?
5. How often do you experience these thoughts?
6. How do you feel when you have these images?
7. What do you do to deal with this?
8. Do you try to ignore or get rid of these images/thoughts and put them out of your mind?
9. Do you tell yourself things or image things to counteract the unpleasant images/thoughts? Do you recognize that these are your own thoughts/images or somebody else put these in your mind?
10. Do you think that these thoughts/images are reasonable or it seems excessive? (to differentiate from psychosis).
11. Have you been criticized by somebody?
12. In order to alleviate obsessions, the patient develops compulsions: Some people are bothered of having to do something over and over again for example: checking, counting, washing hands, praying. Have you experienced one of those? Do you have any rituals that you always have to do in a particular order and if the order is wrong you have to start all over again?
13. Social H/o: How much these obsessions and compulsions affect the patient's every day life?

14. Has it affected your job? marriage? relationship with friends, social life? leisure activities?
15. Does it keep you from completing your daily activities-chores?
16. How much time a day do you spend thinking about this?
17. Stressors in life. Home, work place, education, partner etc.
18. Screen for others: Anxiety disorders, mania, depression, psychosis, hypochondriasis, cognition, and personality disorders.
19. Suicidal ideations and substance abuse.
20. Take a brief PMH, ask about medications, allergies, and ask about family H/o of psychiatric diseases.
21. Open questions to the patient. Ask what the patient think is going on? Expectations?

When you finish, think about:
1. Think about your DDX: Substance induced anxiety disorder or anxiety disorder due to a medical condition, MDD, GAD, specific phobia, body dysmorphic disorder, trichotillomania, schizophrenia, OCD.
2. Explain what OCD is. Address that in 1997, > than 300,000 Canadians were suffering from OCD. Explain the chemical imbalance as a theory and that the patient is "not crazy".
3. Explain what treatments are available nowadays: Psychologic (exposure response prevention, behavior therapy) and medication (SSRIs, clomipramine, benzodiazepines).
4. Explain that even though most patients respond well to the treatment, it may take few weeks for medication to work and the symptoms to be relieved. Also there is a 30% rate of failure.
5. Offer family counseling, support, groups, and flyers.

Panic attack

Case 1: 28 year old man is referred from ER to your office after he was admitted yesterday a few hrs because of chest pain and palpitations.
Case 2: A 25 year old woman is brought by her mother to see you. She has not been able to leave her house in the last 3 months.

1. Open question: What brings you here today? If the patient is hooked with the symptoms, do not minimize them. Everybody is telling him/her that nothing is wrong. However, he/she feels like is going to die. So start asking for how long has this been going on? Last episode? Hospitalizations? Were any studies done? Did anybody mention anxiety? What do you think?

2. How much is this affecting the patient's life? Are you able to function? Work? Leave your house? Sleep? Eat? Family situation? Support?

3. Going back to the pain you have been experiencing, I am going to ask you about some symptoms you may have such as: heart racing, CP, SOB, choking, N/V, diarrhea, dizziness-unsteadiness, fear of going crazy, going to die, numbness, sweating, feeling like in a dream, seeing yourself from outside, the world is unreal. How long does it take from the beginning to the peak of the symptoms? Were you able to anticipate that this is going to happen?

4. Emotional abuse that can reduce self-esteem?

5. Screen the rest of anxiety disorders: (if one +ive analyze deeply)
   Agoraphobia: Do you have difficulties leaving your house, being away from home alone, and crowded places? Are you able to go out with a companion?
   Specific phobias: Are you afraid of animals, blood, flies, and heights.
   Social phobias: Do you have difficulties speaking in public, talking to people (your boss, coworkers).
   GAD: Have you been excessively worrying about something?
   Like something bad is going to happen to you?
   Is it hard for you to stop your worrying?
   Ask about the symptoms: Feeling restless, fidgety, tired easily, problems concentrating, irritable, muscle aches, sleeping problems?
   How long have you been feeling like this (>6 m); how much this affect your life?
   PTSD: Have you had any traumatic experience, event, witnessed, involving serious injury or threatened to death.
   OCD: Have you been experiencing repetitive and unreasonable thoughts?

6. Screening for depression, suicide, psychosis, mania, cognitive (consciousness, memory, orientation and intelligence)

7. PMH: DM, thyroid, HTN, asthma, heart, lung diseases.

8. Medications, allergies, substance abuse.
9. Suicidal attempts, thoughts.
10. ROS.
11. Family H/o: Job performance, relationships, family violence/domestic/sexual/psychological/financial abuse/alcohol involvement/psychiatric diseases/finance, restriction in social activities.
12. Expectations, questions and concerns.

When you finish the station think:

1. That this is a patient-centered interview, so you are going to develop a plan with the patient.
2. Explain what anxiety/panic attack is. There are several kinds of anxiety.
3. Reassure about causes of symptoms.
4. Explain it is treatable. Non-pharmacologic (cognitive behavioral, relaxation).
5. Pharmacologic treatment: SSRI, TCA, buspirone, benzodiazepines.
6. If trigger is identified, work on it.
7. Be aware that 30% of people with anxiety abuse alcohol and substances and also are at risk of suicide.
8. Offer family counseling, support.

Mania

Case 1: Mrs. X is a 26 years old woman who was brought by her husband. He says that she was acting strangely in the last week. She does not have a relevant PMH and did not take any medications or drugs. Interview her. Do not conduct a MMSE.
Case 2: Ms. X is a 30 year old woman who suffers from Bipolar disorder. She came to your office because she has not been feeling well in the last month. Her Dr. is on vacation now. She has been well controlled in Lithium for years.

1.   Keep it cool. The patient is going to push you (talking very fast without stopping) Sit down, call the patient by the name, and ask him/her to sit.
2.   Ask your questions twice if you do not get the first time. Ask 1 question at the time.
3.   Do not raise your voice, do not touch the patient. Establish rapport, create a receptive atmosphere. Be confident and in charge of the interview.
4.   Be flexible, facilitate the interview, use silence, and transitions properly.
5.   Read the paper, project, magazine that she is giving you.
6.   Give consent to what she is doing and comment gently when an activity is excessive.
7.   Start with regular questions related to what the problem is. So you are working in this project very hard? How long have you been working like this? (Mania 7 days, hypomania 4 days). Remember that the patient has a lack of insight. So is not going to realize what is going on.
8.   When into the topic, start with the screening mania: "I can see how much energy you are spending in this project/activity"
9.   Do you feel hyper, like you were high on drugs without taking anything?
10.   Did anything cause you good mood? How long did it last?
11.   How many periods like this have you had?
12.   How about days when you were unusually irritable, and quick to argue or fight? Now I am going to ask you about some other things that you might have been experiencing when feeling euphoric.
13.   Are easily distractible so that any little thing can get you off-track?
14.   Have you engaged in pleasurable activities that have a high potential for painful consequences? (having lot of sex, driving very fast and having tickets from police, spending a lot of many so you have problems with finances.)
15.   Do you feel that you have and special talent", abilities or powers?
16.   Flight of ideas: Do you feel that your thoughts are going very fast and racing in your mind?
17.   Did you start new projects, work more, call friends more?
18.   Do you have to take a shower, eat, and take care of yourself?

19. Did you feel restless so it was hard to sit still?
20. Do you need less sleep than usual in order to feel rested?
21. Talkativeness: Do you feel pressure to talk constantly and people could not understand you?
22. Finances, sexual habits.
23. Energy levels, tickets for driving fast.
24. New projects, not finding time for oneself.
25. Did you feel the opposite bee feeling like this? How long, how bad?
26. Suicide. Always ask; they are at high risk.
27. Screen psychosis: Hallucinations/delusions.
28. If case 2: ask for use of Lithium in detail, increase or decrease in doses, side effects, signs and symptoms of toxicity.
29. Address if she is driving. You should report it to the MOT.
30. Take a brief social H/o: Job, marital status, support, friends, family, and substance abuse.
31. Family H/o: Any body in the family with psychiatric conditions: ADH, Bipolar disorder, cyclothymia, anxiety.

Management:
1. You should negotiate with the patient: Hospitalization is required in acute mania, so explain that you are concerned about his/her not eating, sleeping, taking care of him/herself and offer help. Try to explain the Dx.
2. Explain that we have medications that can help. Suggest she/he should stay in the hospital for a few days and it won't interfere with the project/activities she/he is doing.
3. If the patient's refuse, remember that you can certify him/her (involuntary hospitalization).
4. Your DDxs are: Cyclothymic disorder, mood disorder secondary to substance abuse, medications, and general medical conditions.
5. You should diagnose if it is a "Rapid cycling variant". The treatment is different and the prognostic poorer.

Case 1: Acute mania Case 2: Lithium intoxication

1. Lithium toxicity: Occur when patient get minor illnesses. e. g. Fever, G.I symptoms.
2. Clinical features—Slurred speech, drowsiness, muscle weakness, anorexia, vomiting, diarrhea, ataxia, confusion, bradycardia also thyroid changes.
3. Ideal blood level—2milliequivalents/L.

4. If stopped rapidly can cause withdrawal symptoms. Restarting may not be very effective.
5. A patient taking Li now complaints of losing his artistic talents. Take H/o to see whether that was a symptom of mania/whether the patient was goal directed and achieved success.

Case: 35 yr old male, 1 wk hyperactivity, histrionic, spending spree, bizarre behaviour. Take H/o.

1. Causes of one week of bizarre behaviour: manic episode (bipolar mood disorder), depression, drug-induced (steroids, amphetamines, alcohol), organic (hypothyroidism, frontal lobe tumour, MS, dementia), schizophrenia.
2. Criteria for mania: Increased activity, talkativeness, flight of ideas/racing thoughts, inflated self-esteem, decreased need for sleep, distractibility, pleasurable excesses: reckless driving, spending spree, sexual indiscretions.
3. H/o: Onset, duration, chronology, aggravating and relieving factors (drug use).
4. Is patient a danger to himself or others (suicidal or homicidal)?
5. Does patient have alternating up and down periods, how long do these last?
6. How frequent? Are they cycling faster than before?
7. Ask about sleep, interest, guilt, mood, energy, concentration, appetite/weight, psychomotor, suicide/morbid ideation (positive diagnosis of major depression requires 5 of these over 2 wk period).
8. Paranoia, ideas of reference (thought broadcasting, special messages, mind reading), special powers, magical thinking, secret identity, voices, visual or tactile hallucinations.
9. Current life events, stress, relationship problem, bereavement.
10. Previous psychiatric problems, family H/o of psychiatric disorders, substance abuse, relationship problems, problems at work.
11. Work and relationship histories.
12. Ask about hypothyroidism, adrenal dysfunction, hyper-calcemia, mononucleosis.
13. Medications, drugs, alcohol, smoking, allergies, PMH including psychiatric H/o
14. H/o of abuse. Family H/o, ROS.
15. Mental Status: Appearance, attitude (co-operative?), mood/affect (flat, happy, sad, mad), motor, speech (rate, rhythm, volume, quantity, articulation), thought content (delusions, illusions, hallucinations), thought process (coherent, flight of ideas, logical), insight, intellect.
16. Conduct a MMSE.

Depression

You are likely to feel down during this station due to the environment created by the patient. Address the body language of the patient. Show empathy. Offer napkin if patient cries.

1. SIGEMCAPS
    Sad
    Interest
    Guilty feeling
    Energy levels
    Memory loss
    Concentrating ability.
    Appetite
    Psychomotor agitation/depression
    Suicidal thoughts, plans, attempts.
    How long have you had these? (2 weeks duration is necessary for a diagnosis)
2. I am going to ask you the opposite questions:
    Screen mania: Have you felt hyper, like you were high on drugs?
    Have you felt irritable almost agitated? If (+) continue with the DIGFAST questionnaires.
3. Screening for psychosis:
    Hallucinations: Have you ever seen, heard, felt, smelt something others couldn't, didn't?
    Delusions: Have you ever thought that people talking about you, they want to hurt you? They are out there to get you? Do they want to control you? Can they read your thoughts?
4. Screening for anxiety: Are you an anxious person? Worry about the future? Fear of losing control, any panic attacks?
5. Cognitive screen: COMI—Concentration, orientation, memory and intelligence. MMSE may be necessary. Depression can cause pseudo-dementia.
6. Medications: Ask those that can cause depression, alcohol, withdrawal symptoms.
7. Substance abuse.
8. Personal—Finances, family, domestic violence, education, jobs. Rule out post-partum depression, if patient is a female of child bearing age.
9. Rule out depressed mood after death of near ones.
10. Thyroid diseases, cancers etc.
11. PMH: Thyroid diseases, neurological diseases, psychiatric, hematological, cancer.

12. Social/personal H/o: childhood, family situation, H/o of psychiatric diseases, substance/domestic abuse, education, jobs.
13. Open to the patient's questions.
14. Rule out if the patient is suicidal, also whether the symptoms are due to medications.
15. Any trigger factors? Stressors? e.g. Employment/family/finances/level of functioning of the patient.

When you finish your interview address the following issues
1. Explain to the patient what depression is: "Is a chemical imbalance in the brain that causes your symptoms". Tell the patient that is a common condition nowadays.
2. Your DDxs are going to be: Dementia, Schizophrenia, Schizoaffective disorder, Depression secondary to general medical conditions, medication, substance abuse, Bereavement, adjustment disorder with depressed mood, Anxiety disorders.
3. Explain that you need to run some tests to R/o systemic causes of depression; but still the symptoms can be treated.
4. You should know if the patient is at immediate risk of suicide. If (+) you should involuntary hospitalize the patient. If not and the patient commit suicide, you are liable.
5. Explain the nature of treatment: Always is a combination of a) Psychotherapy (self-insight, psychotherapy) and b) Pharmacologic treatment.
6. Explain what to expect from the treatment, prognosis, and rate of failure.
7. If patient has suicidal ideation, never give medication supply for more than 1 week. They may use it to kill themselves.
8. Give an appointment for the next week, so you can monitor the treatment.
9. Offer to discuss the problem with the family.

Case 1: Depression secondary to medication (anti-hypertensives)
Case 2: Masked depression
Case 3: Atypical depression
Case 4: Postpartum depression
Case 5: MDE secondary to wife's disease

Case: 40 yr old woman, appears sad, requests sleeping pills. Manage.

1. SIGEMCAPS

2. Sleep H/o: Usual requirements, chronology of sleep problems, stressors, sleep hygiene (when, where, regularity, shifts at work, late exercise, meals, alcohol, caffeine, prescription and non-prescription remedies, drugs and medications), sleep latency (time to fall asleep), nocturnal awakening, early morning wakening, daytime somnolence, somnolence while driving, working or during conversation.

3. Anhedonia, guilt, hopelessness, fatigue, mood, concentration, memory, appetite, weight gain or loss, irritability, psychomotor retardation/agitation, anxiety, diurnal variation in mood and activity in the morning, suicidal ideation.

4. Must fully explore suicidal ideation: does the patient intend to harm self, reason for suicidal thoughts, current plan, lethality of plan, access to lethal means, has patient given away prized possessions or written final notes to loved ones, previous attempts.

5. Diagnosis of major depression v/s dysthymia. A diagnosis of dysthymia requires depressed mood for most of the day, more days than not, for at least 2 yrs.

6. A diagnosis of depression cannot be made in the face of bereavement within the past 2 months or drug or alcohol abuse.

7. Mental Status: Appearance, attitude (co-operative), mood/affect (flat, sad, happy, mad), motor, speech (rate, rhythm, volume, quantity, articulation), thought content (delusions, illusions, hallucinations), thought process (coherent, flight of ideas, logical), insight, intellect.

8. Depression: D/d—All other psychiatric disorders/substance abuse/dementia/endocrine-hypothyroidism—DM/adrenal dysfunction. Liver and renal failure/chronic fatigue syndrome/Pernicious anaemia/drug side effects-beta blockes/infectious mononucleosis/menopause/cancer-brain, lung and pancreas/5HT-NA-Dopamine shortage are the causes, substance abuse, relationship problems, problems at work.

9. Drug use, smoking, allergies, PMH including psychiatric H/o and H/o of abuse, family H/o.

10. Treatment of Major Depression: Pharmacotherapy, psychotherapy, family therapy. Start Prozac (fluoxetine) 20 mg every morning, may increase to 40 mg q am after 1 week. 12 weeks and maintenance for 12 months. Takes 2-4 wks to work. Therapeutic dose is 20 to 80 mg. Explain side effects of sleep disturbance, anorgasmia, nausea.

11. Proper sleep hygiene: Regular bed and wake times, avoid daytime naps, regular exercise but not late in the evening, do not use the bed for reading, TV, paperwork, etc, and avoid caffeine, alcohol, and smoking.

12. Recurrence 50% after 1 episode; 90% after 3 episodes.

Mini Mental Status Score

1. Orientation to time (year, month, day)—5
2. Orientation to place (country, province, city)—5
3. Repeat 3 names that I am going to tell (pen, pencil, paper)—3
4. (Keep these 3 names in your head. I will ask them later)
5. Concentration (spell WORLD backwards/Serial 7s from 100)—5
6. Repeat "No ifs ands or buts"—1
7. 3-step command (Take that paper, fold once and put in the floor)—3
8. Write a sentence—1
9. Show 2 objects and ask to name—2
10. Do the written command "Close your eyes" (write and show)—1
11. Copy interlocking pentagons—1
12. Recall the 3 names that I told you to keep in your mind—3
    Total = 30

Anorexia Nervosa

Case: 16 yr old girl brought to the office by a classmate for weight loss over the past 6 months. The classmate is worried about anorexia nervosa. Take H/o and counsel.

1. H/o: Amount of weight lost, time frame, how did patient lose the weight?
2. What is the patient's diet now? Still losing weight?
3. How often does the patient weigh herself? Are you proud of this weight loss?
4. Do you think you need to lose more?
5. Do you admire women who are smaller than you are? Binge eating?
6. Forced post-prandial vomiting, laxative or diuretic abuse, excessive exercise, diet pills?
7. Wearing baggy clothes to conceal "fatness", unable to look at self in a mirror or to be touched by others.
8. Ask about the environment: Is there a problem with expressing conflict openly?
9. Signs of malnutrition: Amenorrhea, sallow skin, rash, easy bruising, dry and sparse hair, lassitude, weakness, anaemia, neurological findings (carpal and tarsal nerve compression, confusion, emotional lability, loss of cortico-spinal vibration and position sense), glossitis, heartburn, teeth erosion, GI bleeding.
10. Counselling: Determine ideal body weight using standard height/weight charts (BMI), ideal is about 20-25 for females.
11. Show the patient her position on the chart.
12. Explain that anorexia nervosa is a modern disease of highly motivated young women. These women exercise extreme control over their bodies, often as a means of sublimating their inability to express conflict at home.
13. Warn patient that excessive weight loss has led to the deaths of many young women who were unable to correct their anorexia. Explain that proper body weight is essential for health and mental function including learning and performing well at school.
14. You understand that the patient may be proud of her weight loss. Being underweight may show a great deal of self control and will power, but being at ideal weight shows more.
15. Invite patient to develop a healthy body image by not equating soft or fatty body areas with overweight. Emphasize that attractiveness and good health depend on a good balance of fatty tissues as well as lean.
16. Contract with the patient to regain at least two pounds each week. Discuss how she will do this.

17. Involve dietician, halt diuretics, laxatives, diet pills, close monitoring of weight, vitals, heart rhythm, and potassium.
18. Arrange follow-up with patient and her family to discuss family dynamics, expression of conflict in the home.

Obesity

Case: An obese person wants to lose weight.

1. Eating frequency, snacking, eating at night, foods eaten, binge eating, guilt about food, concealing eating from others.
2. Calculate daily caloric intake.
3. Alcohol intake, smoking, drug use. Exercise H/o.
4. Associated diseases: Hypothyroidism, DM type II, Cushing's, depression, anxiety disorder, medications (TCA, steroids, OCP), gout, sleep apnoea, cholecystitis, back pain, cardiovascular disease, haemorrhoids, lower limb joint pain and osteoarthritis.
5. Why is seeking help now?
6. Crisis in patient's life, stress, anxiety?
7. Medications, drugs and alcohol, allergies, PMH, family H/o.
8. ROS.
9. O/E: Vitals, calculate BMI = 20-25 for a male and based on frame. (>20% = obese).
10. Cushinoid features: Moon facies, buffalo hump, striae, visual field defects.
11. Fat distribution: Centripetal fat associated with greater heart disease and diabetes risk.
12. Fundoscopy for retinopathy. Cardiopulmonary exam.
13. Signs of hypothyroidism + forgetful, change in personality progressing to psychosis, deep tendon reflexes show slow return phase, leukonychia (whitened nails), orange palms and soles due to carotene deposition, brady-cardia, pericardial effusion, pleural effusions, myxedema (non-pitting edema), carpal and tarsal tunnel nerve compression due to myxedema.
14. Over weight relatives?
15. Counselling: Ideal body weight improves the life. Self-esteem, relationship benefits.
16. Discuss diets tried and why these failed.
17. Fad diets involve unusual or extreme eating patterns and are not designed to be maintained for a lifetime.
18. SSRIs may help loss weight, but when discontinued, regain the weight.
19. Satiety set point which can be reset over time with reduction in caloric intake.
20. Recommend a balanced diet consisting of ordinary foods, with three distinct meals per day of small size.
21. No eating at night and be careful of snacks.

22. Inform patient that he will be hungry as a sign of positive progress on weight loss.
23. Reduce fat to 20% of caloric intake.
24. Calorie requirement: males 10-12 calories/lb; females 8-10 calories/lb.
25. Caloric intake is more important for weight loss than food consumption; reducing fat alone is not sufficient.
26. Exercise as an excuse for overeating and may be dangerous in an obese patient. Recommend mild daily exercise such as 1 hr walk/day.
27. Vigorous exercise can be initiated when weight is lost.

Hysteria

Case: Young woman with tunnel vision. Negative investigations by a neurologist and ophthalmologist. Take H/o. Concerned that her husband has an extramarital affair. Counsel.

1. Visual problem, onset, duration, chronology, functional limitations.
2. Aggravating/relieving factors.
3. Headache, eye pain, nausea, anxiety, palpitations, tremor.
4. Past H/o of eye problems, paralysis, numbness, abdominal pain.
5. Problems at work, home, with relationships?
6. What is the support system in life?
7. Depression and sleep H/o.
8. Psychiatric problems in the past?
9. Medications, drug and alcohol use, allergies, PMH, family H/o.
10. ROS.
11. Validate the patient's feelings and then counsel.
12. Even though specialists didn't find anything wrong with the vision, does not mean that there is no medical problem. So it is important to stick with one doctor.
13. People who are faced with marital infidelity activate a defence mechanism which gives them time to adjust, and which is not under conscious control.
14. This helps the patient to get support from others. This is a normal reaction.
15. These include paralysis, numbness, pain, inability to speak, visual problems.
16. Discussion with the patient's husband about fidelity is required.
17. If both partners are willing, a consultation with a marital therapist.
18. Consolidate a support network of parents, friends.
19. Consider depression, sleep or anxiety medications.
20. Arrange follow-up with both partners.

Section 8

Obstetrics and Gynaecology

Vaginal bleeding
Vaginal discharge
Amenorrhoea
Counseling oral contraceptive devices
Counseling hormone replacement therapy
Pregnancy counsel
Infertility
Pre-eclampsia
Therapeutic abortion
Cancer Cervix—counseling

Vaginal bleeding

Case 1: 35 years old woman c/o of vaginal spotting 3 weeks.
Case 2: 32 years old woman c/o abdominal pain and irregular periods.
Case 3: 45 years osld woman c/o because of irregular bleeding.
Case 4: 60 years old woman c/o because of vaginal bleeding.

1. OCD: since when? Is it getting worse? Why? Ask symptoms of hypovolemia.
2. How many pads/day (>6 is serious), clots, LMP (how long, how many days apart, regular, painful cycles).
3. Identify the pattern of bleeding: (amount/color/timing)
   a. Menorrhagia = >7 days or > 80 ml
   b. Hypomenorrhea = Less bleeding < ml
   c. Polymenorrhea = <21 days for a cycle
   d. Oligomenonhea = > 35 days for a cycle
   e. Metronhagia = irregular intervals
   f. Menometrorrhagia = Increased amount and irregular intervals
4. Ask about post-coital bleeding Age of menarche/menopause.
5. Analyze pain: PQRST. How bad is it? Did you miss work because of it? PMS.
6. Endometriosis: Is it getting worse over the years, begin in the middle of the cycle, low back pain before the periods, pain going to the rectum.
7. Menopause: Hot flashes, vaginal dryness, dysuria, mood swings, insomnia, dyspareunia, fatigue.
8. Endometriosis: N/V, dyspareunia, pain with bowel movements, urination, infertility, miscarriages.
9. Cervical Ca: Post-coital bleeding, fatigue, dyspareunia, bone pain, back pain, bladder/bowel symptoms, D&C, pelvic heaviness.
10. Endometrial ca: Same as cervical.
11. DUB: Absent PMS (anovulatory stage), previous irregular bleeding (scanty or heavy), infertility, hirsutism, obesity.
12. RF for endometriosis: Nulliparity, age between 30-40, family H/o, heavy periods > 8 days, short cycles.
13. RF for cervical ca: HPV, multiparity, smoking, HIV, early intercourse, multiple partners, low socioeconomic status.
14. RF for endometrial ca: Unopposed estrogen (PCO, late menopause/early menarche, obesity, nulliparity).
15. H/o of breast, liver, ovary colon cancers, pelvic irradiation, tamoxifen, DM.

16. QB/GYN H/o: GTPAL, PAPs, mamograms, STD, procedures, surgeries, treatment for infertility.
17. BCP, HRT, Tamoxifen, HIV, sexual H/o.
18. PMH: HTN, DM, kidney, thyroid, liver, bleeding disorders, trauma.
19. Medications: BCP, HRT, tamoxifen, aspirin, warfarin.
20. Allergies.
21. Social: Alcohol, smoking, drugs, occupation.
22. Family H/o: Gynec. cancers.

Case: 60 yr old female with bloody vaginal discharge. Take H/o.

1. Onset of bleeding, frequency, estimate quantity (# of pads), colour, consistency of discharge, associated pain, vaginal discomfort, cramping.
2. Post coital and rectal bleeding.
3. Weight loss, night sweats, fatigue.
4. Age of menarche, age of menopause, age of first sexual activity.
5. Use of hormonal replacement therapy, which preparation?
6. H/o of fibroids, reproductive tract cancers, last Pap smear, pregnancy H/o.
7. Medications, drugs/alcohol, smoking.
8. PMH, surgical H/o, family H/o, ROS.

Case: 30 yr old woman with vaginal bleeding at 30 wks of gestation. Take H/o. Give DDx. Order investigations.

1. GTPAL, weeks of gestation.
2. Onset of bleeding, duration, estimate quantity (# of pads soaked), colour and consistency of blood.
3. Associated fever, chills, abdominal discomfort, contractions, fetal movement, light-headedness, last sexual intercourse (may cause spotting due to friable cervix).
4. Problems with previous pregnancies, problems in this pregnancy, medical visits to this point, investigations done.
5. Associated abdominal trauma (accident or abuse), drug use (cocaine), father and mother's blood type.
6. Medications, alcohol, smoking, PMH, family H/o, ROS.
7. DDx: placenta previa (placenta covers internal os of cervix—the most common cause of painless bleeding in the 3rd trimester), premature rupture of membranes, abruptio placenta (separation of placenta from uterine wall—usually painful), vasa previa (fetal bleed due to root vessels of umbilical cord overlying the cervical os—extremely dangerous to the fetus).

8. Other causes: Uterine rupture, coagulopathy (DIC), molar gestation, vaginal tear, vaginal infection, cervical polyp, cervicitis, cervical cancer.
9. Investigations: Maternal visits, CBC, INR/PTT, fibrinogen, type and crossmatch if bleeding is severe, Rh status (may need Rhogam gamma globulin to prevent formation of antibodies against fetal blood if mother is Rh negative and father is Rh positive).
10. Fetal monitor, fetal u/s, maternal monitoring, IV access, pelvic speculum and manual exam with digital cervical exam (Do these only after U/S—can cause further bleeding in previa).
11. Apt test for fetal hemoglobin in vaginal blood, test maternal blood for presence and amount of fetal hemoglobin (determines amount of Rhogam required to neutralize fetal blood antigenicity).

Case 1: Cervical ca.
Case 2: Endometriosis
Case 3: DUB
Case 4: Endometrial ca.

Vaginal discharge

Case 1: 22 years old woman is coming to see you because of vaginal discharge.
Case 2: 27 yr. old in ER complaining of vaginal D/c, fever and abdominal pain.
Case 3: 20 years old woman is coming to see you because she presents with the 3ʳᵈ
vaginal infection in this year.

1. OCD: first time? Has this happen before? How many times in a year?
2. Analyze the D/C: Relation with period: pre/postmenstrual, color, odor, amount, consistency, does it smell more after intercourse?
3. Analyze pain: PQRST.
4. Associated symptoms: Itchiness, dysuria, dyspareunia, bleeding, fever, chills, joint pain, skin rash, warts on the genitalia, adenopathies.
5. Ask about sexual partner's symptoms.
6. Risk factors PID: Young age, IUD, previous PID, multiple sexual partners, partner with symptoms, soon after LMP and intercourse.
7. RFs chlamydia and gonococci, infertility. OB/GYN H/o.
8. LMP. Do you think you may be pregnant?
9. Previous PIDs, vaginal D/C, treatment D/C.
10. GTPAL, ectopics, tubo-ovarian Sxs, STD, HIV, PAPs, HPV, genital warts, endometriosis, cancer, fibroids.
11. Take a sexual H/o as well H/o of IUD.
12. PMH: Apendicitis or pelvic surgeries, DM, HTN.
13. Medications: BCP, antibiotics, steroids, allergies.
14. Smoking, alcohol, drugs.
15. Social: Occupation-Prostitute? (Ask after offering confidentiality), travels.

When you finish think about:
1. DDx?
2. You need to examine the patient. What signs are you going to look for?
3. Do you think that this patient needs admission? Criteria admission in PID?
4. Studies to be done? Wet swabs, U/S, HIV, STDs.
5. Do you have to report this case?
6. What treatment are you going to implement? If ambulatory, when do you want to see this patient again? What about the partner?
7. If PID is the Dx, what are the chances of infertility after 1/2/3 episodes?
8. If repetitive vaginal candidiasis, which conditions would you think about?

Case I: Trichomoniasis
Case 2: Tubo-ovarian abscess
Case 3: DM/HIV related candidiasis.

Case: 19 yr old female with a vaginal discharge. Take H/o. Q: Give three possible diagnoses. What investigations would differentiate these?

1. Description of discharge, onset, chronology, previous episodes, volume, colour, consistency, odour, and timing (related to menses?).
2. Associated symptoms: Pain including abdominal, burning, fever, itch, dyspareunia, dysuria, urgency, frequency, aggravating and relieving factors.
3. Sexual H/o: Number of past and present partners, gender, type of contraception (condoms?), possibility of pregnancy.
4. Past H/o of STDs. Obs/Gyn H/o.
5. Pregnancies, abortions/miscarriages, births, PAP smears normal?
6. Menstrual pattern.
7. Medications especially antibiotics, OCP, other drug use, allergies.
8. PMH including diabetes. Family H/o, ROS.
9. Causes of vaginitis: Candidiasis, bacterial vaginosis, trichomonas infection (gonorrhea and chlamydia can cause cervicitis, PID and urethritis, but do not cause vaginitis).
10. Investigations: Speculum exam, swab and culture, saline slide microscopy and KOH whiff test (add KOH to vaginal secretions on a slide).
11. Candidiasis: inflamed appearance, lumpy white discharge, spores and pseudohyphae seen under microscope. Rx: miconazole vaginal suppository.
12. Bacterial vaginosis: Non-inflamed, thin grey secretions, clue cells under microscope (epithelial cells with obscured borders due to adherence of bacteria), fishy odour on KOH test. Rx: metronidazole 500 mg po BID x 7 days (in pregnancy use Amoxicillin 500 mg TID x 7 days).
13. Trichomonas: Inflammation, frothy yellow-green discharge, motile trichomonads seen under microscope. Rx: metronidazole 2 g x 1 or 500 mg po BID X 7 days (in pregnancy use clotrimazole vaginal suppositories).

Amenorrhea

Case 1: 27 years old woman with 3 missed periods.
Case 2: 28 years old obese woman with irregular periods.
Case 3: 25 years old woman with a 5 month H/o of amenorrhea.

1. Start with the OCD: Have you ever missed a period before?
2. Analyze the pattern of bleeding: Amenorrhea? oligoamenorrhea? spotting? post-coital spotting?
3. OB/GYN H/o: Periods in detail, LMP, characteristics, always irregular? onset, menarche.
4. Signs of ovulation: PMS, dysmenorrhea, mittelschmerz
5. GTPAL, last pregnancy, lactation, sexual H/o.
6. D/C, treatments infertility.
7. Rule out post-pill amenorrhoea. Amenorrhea might continue up to 6 months after stopping OCP.
8. Pregnancy: Breast tenderness, N/V, fatigue, skin changes.
9. Do you think you may be pregnant?
10. Ovarian failure: Hot flashes, vaginal dryness, fatigue, depression, dysuria.
11. PCO: Obesity, hirsutism, infertility, irregular bleeding.
12. Hypotalamus-hypophysis: Anorexia, weight loss, stress, headache, visual changes, galactorrhea.
13. Hypothalamic take a HEEADDS interview.
14. Pituitory—milk discharge from the nipples and headache. Investigate with prolactin; Also ask about involvement in motor vehicle accident.
15. Uterus—recent D&C, hysterectomy, Asherman's syndrome.
16. Hypothyroidism: Cold intolerance, weight gain, skin changes, constipation, goiter.
17. PMH: Thyroid, DM, HTN, Autoimmune disease (assoc. with ovarian failure), and chronic diseases.
18. ROS—Thyroid, kidney, lung, heart.
19. Abdominal surgeries, depression.
20. Medications: BCP, Psychiatric medication, methyldopa, antidepressants.
21. Allergies, smoking, alcohol, drugs.
22. Social: Occupation, stress, diet, hobbies (runners, dancers), home situation.
23. Family H/o: PCO, premature ovarian failure, brain tumors.
24. Key points: Start thinking from head to below. Hypothalamo-pituitory: anorexia, weight loss, stress, headache, visual changes; Thyroid: hypothyroidism; Ovary: PCO obesity, hirsuitism, infertility; Menopause; Uterus: preganacy.

25. Endogenous testosterones are DHEA and DHEAS. These are good for bone density and libido. High dose of oestrogens in ORT may reduce them.
26. Investigations: Beta HCG, prolactin, LH, FSH, estrogen, progesterone, TSH, DHEAS, testosterone, progesterone challenge test and head CT.

Case 1: Post-pill amenorrhea
Case 2: PCO
Case 3: Prolactinoma.

Case: 7 wks pregnant with lower abdominal pain and vaginal bleeding. Take H/o. H/o previous spontaneous abortion at 6 wks gestation. Give D/d. What 3 findings on vaginal exam would confirm this diagnosis?

1. Threatened abortion = any uterine bleeding or cramping in the first 20 wks of gestation.
2. Inevitable abortion = intolerable pain or bleeding for 1 week, cervix open. Life threatening to the mother.
3. Incomplete abortion = membranes ruptured, part of products of conception passed, cervix open.
4. Complete Abortion = uterus empty, cervix closed. 20-30% of pregnancies have uterine bleeding or cramping in the first 20 weeks. Half of these abort.
5. Most spontaneous abortions are associated with an abnormal fetus.
6. H/o: Patient ID (name, age, occupation), GTPAL, weeks of gestation.
7. Onset of bleeding, duration, estimate quantity (number of pads soaked), last time had sexual intercourse (friable cervix), colour and consistency of blood, associated fever, chills, abdominal discomfort, light headedness.
8. Problems with previous pregnancies, problems in this pregnancy, medical visits to this point, investigations done.
9. Associated abdominal trauma (accident or abuse), drug use (cocaine), father and mother's blood type, medications, alcohol, smoking, PMH (diabetes, lupus).
10. Family H/o, ROS. DDx: Threatened abortion, incomplete abortion, non-uterine bleeding source (vaginal, cervical, vulvar).
11. Most likely Dx: Incomplete abortion.
12. Findings which would confirm incomplete abortion: Ruptured membranes, products of conception passed, cervix dilated.

Case: Young female with secondary amenorrhea for 6 months. Take H/o. What investigations would you order? Give a D/d. What is the most likely diagnosis, what results would confirm this diagnosis?

1. Age of menarchy, regularity of previous menses, flow, duration, accompanying cramps, bloating, psychic disturbance.
2. Headache, visual field disturbance (for sellar tumour).
3. Signs of virlization: Increased quantity and coarseness of body hair and facial hair, acne, increased sexual drive, increased muscle bulk.
4. Galactorrhea? Diet H/o: Has patient lost/gained weight recently?
5. Thyroid symptoms: Energy levels, emotional lability/depression, cold intolerance, or feels hot, jumpiness.
6. Exercise H/o: Is patient engaging in vigorous exercise such as running?
7. Sexual H/o: Contraception. Is pregnancy a possibility?
8. Medications, drugs, and alcohol use, smoking.
9. PMH with surgical H/o, family H/o, ROS.
10. Investigations: $Beta-hCG, TSH, serum LH, FSH, serum prolactin, serum testosterone, sex-hormone binding globulin (SHBG), DHEA-S, progesterone trial for future uterine bleeding (indicated functional endometrium).
11. DDx: Pregnancy, polycystic ovary syndrome (Stein-Leventhal syndrome), hypothalamic dysfunction, excessive exercise, stress, weight loss, adrenal hyperfunction (e.g. Cushing's), thyroid dysfunction, prolactinoma, hypopituitarism.
12. Most likely Dx: Polycystic ovary is confirmed by elevated LH, low or normal FSH with well estrogenized vaginal mucosa, increased serum androgens, ovarian cysts seen on ultrasound.

Counseling about birth control pills (BCP)

Case: 20 years old woman comes to talk to you about the "Pill"

1. Start your interview by asking the patient if she is only interested on the pill". Would she like to know also about other contraceptive methods?
2. Ask about why she decided to ask the pill now, previous experiences, how long, why did she stop? What contraceptive method was she using so far?
3. Take a brief OB/GYN H/o: Is there a possibility that the patient could be pregnant? LMP, regular or not, H/o of STD, HIV, PID, D/C, Pap smear, GTPAL. H/o of any problems with previous pregnancies.
4. Take a brief sexual H/o: How long has the patient been sexually active? # of partners, close relationship, partner in good health, partner's support with regards to BCP.
5. PMH of medications, allergies, alcohol, smoking (BCP and smoking is not a good combination), drugs, migraine, fibroids, diabetes, thromboembolic disease, heart problems, cancer, liver disease.
6. Contraindications BCP: Absolute: pregnancy, undiagnosed vaginal bleeding, active liver disease, breast cancer, H/o of DVT/PE. Relative: DM, smoking, migraine, MI, breastfeeding.
7. Start counseling by explaining how the pill works (prevent ovulation and makes the mucus thick). Think about what kind of pill would be beneficial to this patient (combined E/P v/s mini pill).
8. Explain the benefits: Very low rate of failure (<2%) if taken properly, regular/light periods, less anemia, protects against: PID, osteoporosis, PMS, dysmenorrhea, breast cysts, endometriosis, and ectopic pregnancy.
9. Place package in an obvious location to help you remember.
10. One should take 1 tablet every day: what to do if you forget 1/2/3 tablets. Miss 1—Take 2 next day; Miss 2—a) Take 2 each for next 2 days and use an alternative method until the next period. b) But it is in the 3rd week of cycle, discard that pack and start another pack + supplement with another contraceptive method.
11. How to take it: Explain 21 pills of hormones + 7 pills of iron = 28d. Better to take it at the same time every day. When to start (1st day of the period=protection right away, or 1st Sunday after. Should use condom during the first month). Explain that she will have the period every month.
12. Minipill = projesterone alone.
13. If bleeding and spotting on day 1 to 9—change OCP to one with more oestrogen; if bleeding and spotting from day 10 to 21—change OCP with more projesterone.

14. Side effects: mild bleeding in1st 2 months, N/V, breast pain, mild wt gain.
15. Warning signs: CP, SOB, severe headache, vision changes, epistaxis.
16. If you have to take another medication any reason or N/V/diarrhea = notify your F.P.
17. Also depot injections for 3 years and implants for 5 years are available.
18. Explain that you have to do some tests before starting: P/E + pelvic exam, labs, PAP smear.
19. Explain that BCP does not protect against STD or HIV.

Counseling about hormone replacement therapy (HRT)

Case: 55 years old woman comes to talk to you regarding HRT.

1. Start asking the patient why did she decide to come?
2. Information regarding HRT? Previous experiences? Anybody close in HRT?
3. Ask about general health issues: Signs of menopause, signs of osteoporosis, and signs of CAD.
4. RF—OP, CAD.
5. Brief OB/GYN H/o: Physiologic or surgical menopause.
6. Contraindications for HRT: Vaginal bleeding, breast/uterus/liver cancer, active thromboembolic disease. Relative: migraine, HTN, smoking, stroke, fibroids.
7. PMH of relevance.
8. Start your counseling by explaining what menopause means. Explain if she would be a good candidate to HRT according to her risks.
9. Benefits: People feel healthier, look younger and make the bones thicker. Benefits proved are: decrease in the symptoms of menopause, decrease the progression of osteoporosis, and decreases the chances of Alzheimer disease, in regards to CAD: HERS showed not benefits in secondary prevention, may be some benefits primary prevention.
10. Risk of HRT: Increase in the incidence of breast ca: lifetime risk in general population is 9%, with HRT is 13%, also endometrial ca if not progesterone. So each time she presents with bleeding, a uterine sample is necessary.
11. Why most women do not go HRT: Fear to gain weight, breast ca, bleeding.
12. Options: Long-term treatments, short-time, go alternatives. Is your personal decision.
13. How to take it: Cyclic, continuous, patch, cream.
14. Warning signs: Heavy bleeding, SOB, CP, severe headache, breast lumps.
15. You can comment in other options if the patient wants to know: Calcium, exercise, diet, biphosphonates, and raloxifene.
16. Offer flyers, magazines, info. Be open to her questions. The decision should not be made today. Set up another appointment if necessary.

Pregnancy Counsel

Case: 37 yr old well G1P0 female, 9 wks pregnant. Manage.

1. Planned pregnancy? Stable relationship?
2. Previous pregnancies, abortions. Provisions for care of child when born?
3. Smoking (prepared to quit?), alcohol (no alcohol during pregnancy), illicit drugs.
4. Diet, exercise, medications (avoid during pregnancy, including over-the-counter).
5. Diabetes, family H/o of inherited disorders.
6. Heart disease, circulatory problems, renal disease, hypertension.
7. Menstrual H/o, regularity of cycles, how long has patient not used contraception.
8. Last menstrual period, EDC, any morning sickness?
9. Vaginal bleeding? PMH, surgical H/o, family H/o, ROS.
10. Physical: Vitals, weight, height, palpation of neck and thyroid glands.
11. Fundoscopic exam, check lid lag, reflexes, cardiopulmonary exam, breast exam.
12. Abdominal exam, palpate uterus, measure symphysis-umbilicus distance.
13. Doppler for fetal heart (likely undetectable until 10 weeks).
14. Vaginal bimanual exam and speculum exam (cervix should be closed).
15. Pap smear (use speculum not brush in os), swab cervix for cultures.
16. Investigations: CBC, lytes, INR/PTT, BUN, Cr, urinalysis, ECG, blood type, Rh factor, VDRL and Hep B screen, rubella antibody, serum folate. Urine dip, microscopy and culture. TB skin test if patient is from an endemic area, genetic testing as indicated on H/o for sickle cell in blacks. Alpha fetoprotein at 15-16 wks, amniocentesis or chorionic villous sampling should be offered given patient's age. Fetal ultrasound.
17. Counselling: Discuss risks of Down's syndrome due to maternal age, value of fetal genetic testing.
18. Recommend daily pregnancy vitamin preparations, milk and healthy diet.
19. Do not increase food intake dramatically—excessive weight gain not recommended. 2-3 lb per month for a total of 25-20 lb gain in weight is ideal.
20. Do not diet during pregnancy. Continue normal activities and customary exercise.
21. No alcohol, no smoking, no medications of any kind unless discussed with MD.
22. Control morning sickness with small meals and bland foods.
23. Lying on side decreases swelling and discomfort.

24. Hemorrhoids, backache, heartburn, increased vaginal discharge are common.
25. Follow-up every 4 wks until 32 weeks, then increase to q 2 wks until 36 weeks then q weekly.
26. Call if concerns or troubling symptoms, especially abdominal pain, vaginal bleeding, persistent headache, illness or infection.

Infertility

Case: 27 year old woman comes to see you because she was trying to get pregnant without success.

1. Start your interview by making sure that this is a case of infertility (unprotected sex a year).

2. Show concern about the patient's desire to get pregnant w/o success. Ask if the partner is also involved and supportive towards the situation.

3. OCD: How long have you been trying to get pregnant? Did you have other relationships before this one? Any proved pregnancy? What about your partner? Does he have any children?

4. Start with the patient's OB/GYN H/o: When was your LMP, How long is the period? How many days apart? Painful? Regular? Age of menarche? Inter-menstrual bleeding? Post-coital bleeding? Have you ever been pregnant? GTPAL, complications (C-sections, infections, Rh group), STD, PID, HIV, pap smears, fertility treatments.

5. Associated symptoms
   Ovulation: PMS, dysmenorrhea, breast tenderness, Mittleischmerz.
   Thyroid disease: weight changes, cold/heat intolerance, goiter.
   H-P disease: vision problems, galactorrhea, headaches, stress, exercise.
   Anorexia nervosa: weight loss, muscle cramps, dentition problems.
   Tubal factors: Vaginal D/C, previous Sx, gynec. procedures, IUD and PID.
   PCO: obesity, hirsutism, DM.
   Endometriosis: painful periods, abnormal bleeding pattern.
   Ovarian failure: hot flushes, vaginal dryness, mood swings, symptoms of autoimmune diseases.

6. Take a sexual H/o in detail: Average of sexual intercourses in a month. Unprotected? Spermicidal creams? Vaginal penetration = fluid leaking after the intercourse? Dyspareunia? Technique, Bleeding? Does your husband achieve normal erections? Ejaculation? Anxiety? Do you check the temperature by BBT?

7. PMH: Thyroid problems, congenital abnormalities, DM, HTN, irradiations, Cancers, Medications, Psychiatric, BCP, Allergies, smoking, alcohol, drugs.

8. Social H/o: Occupation, exposure to toxins, diet, exercise, marital situation, partner support.

9. Family H/o: infertility.

10. Partner H/o: age, previous children, occupation (driver, cook, toxin contact), alcohol, smoking, drugs, DM, HTN, impotence, prostate problems,

mumps, TB, STD, HIV, traumas, Sx, varicocele, medications: ASA. Any semen analysis before?

11. Counseling: Explain that the studies involved in approaching infertility can be easy and quick at the beginning and some others also bothersome and time-consuming. Are you ready that? Normal rate of success = 60% first year, 80% in second (40% male factors and 40% female factors and 20% unknown).

12. Explain about modifying simple factors: Stop smoking, alcohol, coffee, drugs, obesity (both partners). Educate with regards to BBT, sexual intercourse or other simple factors.

13. Definition of realistic expectations: Unmet expectations are the greatest source of dissatisfaction infertile couples. Encourage the couple to work together. Deal with emotions and anxiety.

14. Outline the studies:

15. Pelvic exam, PAP smear.

16. Semen analysis: Your partner should do the test, probably more then once.

17. Blood work: Progesterone, prolactin, LH/FSH, TSH, testosterone, DHEAS, estrogen, U/S, swabs (C + G), post-coital test.

18. FSH/LH ratio >2 means PCOD; If both low—pituitary cause; If both high—premature ovarian failure.

19. Projesterone challenge test—Give projesterone for 10 days. Stop. If bleeding occrurs then ostrogen is normal.

20. If no source is found, consider referral to fertility clinic.

21. Clomiphene, IVF, tuboplasty and sperm washing.

22. Adoption is also an option.

Pre-eclampsia

Case: Pregnant woman, 36 wks gestation, has proteinuria and BP 130/85 (pre-gestational BP 110/65). Manage.

1. Hypertension may be pregnancy-induced, or pre-existing hypertension can be worsened by pregnancy.
2. Pre-eclampsia is pregnancy-induced or worsened hypertension (systolic BP increased by 30 mmHg and diastolic by 15 mmHg) with renal impairment or edema.
3. Eclampsia is pre-eclampsia with CNS involvement, usually consciousness and seizures.
4. Other end organs may be affected, particularly the liver and placenta. May progress to death through multi-organ failure.
5. Counselling: You have pre-eclampsia. Define as above.
6. Condition is common, 5% of the pregnant population, more common in first pregnancies. Cause is poorly understood, seems to involve secretion of a substance by the placenta which raises blood pressure. Severity varies. Risks for mother: end organ dysfunction (kidneys, liver, brain), loss of pregnancy, death.
7. Risks for fetus: Malnutrition, hypoxia, low birth weight, incomplete maturation, death. Overall treatment strategy is to slow progression of hypertension until the baby can be delivered. Delivery is curative.
8. Management: Initial exam and investigations: vitals, body weight, examine for edema, check for RUQ tenderness, reflexes. CBC, lytes, Cr, urinalysis with microscopy, 24 hr urine protein, LFTs, INR/PTT, FHR, non-stress test, biophysical profile (USG with 5 criteria).
9. Follow-up: Daily BP, daily weight, daily reflexes, fetal movement counts at home (if patient lives reasonably close to a hospital and can get transportation fast), frequent follow-up visits for blood work, urinalysis and fetal monitoring, bed rest (preferably left side).
10. Instruct patient on worsening signs: Rapid weight gain, liver pain, visual disturbance, persistent headache, drowsiness or seizures.
11. Delivery: Early hospital admission (@ 36 weeks) for close monitoring and administration of IV $MgSO_4$ 4 g if signs of CNS involvement are present (hyper-reflexia, decreased consciousness, seizure).
12. Possible induction of early delivery or C-section. When you talk to the patient never say "We will induce delivery". Never use the word "induce".

13. Consider methyldopa if delivery is not imminent or IV hydralazine if delivery is imminent to decrease BP after conservative measures tried. (Diuretics and salt or fluid restriction not useful and may be harmful).

Therapeutic abortion

Case: First year university student, 9 weeks pregnant, considering abortion. Take H/o and counsel. Findings: tearful, guilty, sleep disturbance, has not engaged social supports.

1. Combine a pregnancy H/o with a social H/o and a screen for depression.
2. Past medical H/o, family H/o, medications, drugs, and review of systems).
3. Pregnancy: GTPAL (# of gestations, term pregnancies, premature births, abortions, live children).
4. H/o of problems, if any, with previous pregnancies. Current pregnancy: establish gestational age by LMP. If periods are regular, the gestational age is the number of weeks from the LMP less 2 weeks. Ask about use of alcohol, smoking, drugs, maternal illnesses during the pregnancy (particularly diabetes, rubella, toxoplasmosis, herpes, CMV, thyroid dysfunction, hypertension, hypercoagulation). Use of birth control, if any. Past medical H/o, family H/o of pregnancy-related problems, medications.
5. Social: Status of any relationships at present including the relationship with the child's father. Social supports (family, friends, boyfriend). Do they know? Are they helping?
6. Employment/financial/educational status of the patient. Does she feel prepared to raise a child?
7. Psychiatric: How does the patient feel about this decision? How is she coping? Cover mnemonic for major depression (SIGEMCAPS: sleep, interest, guilt, energy, concentration, appetite, psychomotor, suicide). Positive diagnosis of major depression requires five of these over a 2 week period, one of the five must be a loss of interest or depressed mood.
8. Counselling: Base advice on problems identified on the obtained H/o. (Note that it is always advisable while counselling to make empathetic statements…"This must be hard for you.")
9. Health while pregnant: Recommend abstinence from harmful agents (alcohol, smoking) while pregnant, and use of medications only after consulting with a physician, treatment for pregnancy-related illnesses as above, and healthy eating habits.
10. Social Supports: Discuss the importance of engaging social supports and consider a visit with both the patient and the partner or other supporting person.
11. Abortion: Provide information on local abortion services.

12. Make the patient aware that the gestational age limit after which many practitioners will not perform an elective abortion in Canada is 20 weeks, but that this is a late limit and her decision should be made sooner.
13. Inform the patient that further advice is available from private gynaecologists who perform abortions and counsellors at elective abortion centres.
14. Offer to refer the patient is she wishes.
15. Depression management: Normalize the patient's depressed mood in view of her circumstances.
16. If there is evidence of major clinical depression, arrange close follow-up to monitor for suicidal ideation, refer to psychiatry. Do not prescribe medications at this time (because of the pregnancy).

Cancer Cervix—counselling

1. Hysterectomy at different stages of Ca Cx depends on the patient's desire for children in future. Therefore, different stages of Ca Cx are kept as a station.
2. Grading of Ca Cx—Corresponding grading of 2 systems.

Atypical squamous cells of undetermined significance (ASCUS)	Squamous atypia of unknown significance.
Low grade squamous intraepithelial Lesion (LGSIL)	HPV atypia or mild dysplasia Cervical intraepithelial neoplasia (CIN I)
High grade SIL (HGSIL)	CIN II and CIN III
	Ca in situ
	Squamous cell carcinoma

Rx:

    a. CIN I (LGSIL)—observe with regular cytology, colposcopy if + on 2 consecutive smears, if progressive-excise with laser/cryotherapy/cone biopsy.

    b. CIN II and III (HGSIL)—laser, cryotherapy, cone excision, Hysterectomy for CIN III—If no desire for future child bearing.

    c. Stage IA—Abdominal hysterectomy, cervical conization if future fertility desired.

    d. Stage IB—Radical hysterectomy, pelvic lymphadenectomy, ovaries spared, Radiotherapy if >4 cm.

    e. Stage 2, 3, 4—Radiotherapy.

3. If this case appear for counselling, it will be better if you can draw a picture of the uterus and cervix and explain.
4. Keep the picture towards the patient's side, so that she can see it promptly.

Section 9

Surgery

Abdominal pain
Delirium tremens
Lymph node enlargement
Black eye
Wound suture
Wrist joint examination
Hematuria
Dysphagia
Back Pain
Carpel tunnel syndrome
Solitary lung nodule
Ankle injury
Disc herniation

Abdominal Pain

Case1. 30 yr old man with hematemesis and abdominal pain in the ER. BP: 80/50.
Give orders to nurse.
Case2. 23 yr old female with 24 hr abdominal pain. Perform focussed P/E.
Findings: peritoneal signs, point tenderness at McBurney's point. Give a DDx, order
investigations. What further H/o would help confirm diagnosis?

1. P/E with pelvic manual and speculum exam.
2. Check for pain with cervical motion (seen in PID), pain on palpation of ovaries, mass, cervical discharge.
3. DDx: Appendicitis, ovarian cyst, rupture or ovarian torsion, mittelschmertz, ectopic pregnancy (life threatening), hepatitis, cholecystitis, gastroenteritis, peptic ulcer, PID, UTI, pyelonephritis, kidney stone, inflammatory bowel disease, intestinal obstruction due to volvulus or IBD.
4. Investigations: Abdominal x-ray 3 views, abdominal-pelvic ultrasound, CBC, lytes, urea, Cr, INR/PTT, glucose, b-HCG, urinalysis, stool for occult blood, cervical swabs for culture and Pap smear.
5. If OR is an emergency, type and cross for 2 units PRBCs, CXR.
6. Further H/o: A H/o of gradual onset vague periumbilical of LLQ pain migrating to a sharper, more localized pain in the RLQ over several hours associated with nausea, anorexia, and controlled by still fetal posture suggests appendicitis.

Case: 62 yr old female with LLQ pain. Perform P/E. Findings: low grade fever, some
abdominal distension, LLQ tenderness without rigidity, poorly defined LLQ mass.
Abdominal series shows multiple air/fluid levels. Describe. Give DDx with most likely
diagnosis. Order further investigations.

1. P/E and abdominal X-ray. Manual and speculum exam of the pelvis.
2. Check for pain with cervical motion (PID), pain on palpation of the ovaries, mass, cervical discharge.
3. DDx: Diverticulitis, diverticular abscess, constipation with obstruction, GI malignancy with perforation, gallstone ileus, obstruction due to volvulus (usually RLQ pain), Crohn's, mesenteric ischemia or infarct, ovarian tumour, PID, uterine perforation.
4. Most likely diagnosis: Diverticulitis
5. Investigations: Abdominal/pelvic CT (U/S if CT unavailable), stool for occult blood, urinalysis, cervical swabs and pap, CBC, lytes, BUN, Cr,

INR/PTT, glucose, for possible pre-op: ECG, CXR, type and cross 4 units PRBCs.

6. Even if you know the diagnosis from the given information, do a systematic H/o taking and P/E including the following.

7. OCD—PQRST—nausea—vomiting—constipation—diarrhea—hematochezia—hematemesis—melena—urinary   symptom—fever—wt. changes—anorexia—NSAIDS—smoke—alcohol; Gynec & Obs—menstrual; O/E: writhing—obstruction; still—peritonitis; do a digital rectal exam.

8. Investigations: CBC and differential; BUN, Cr, amylase, lipase, bilirubin, liver enzymes, coagulation, toxic screen, x-ray abdo, gas under diaphragm, ultrasound for GB and gynecology, CT scan, unine analysis, fecal occult blood, endoscopy and H.pylori.

Black Eye

Case: Young mother with black eye, hit by her boyfriend. Manage.

1. Warning signs of domestic violence: Obsessive partner; need to control the victim by controlling money, restrictions on going out and not allowing to see certain people.
2. Social isolation. Threats and verbal abuse aimed at decreasing self esteem of victim.
3. Cycle of violence followed by remorse, followed by increased violence.
4. Risk Factors for DV: Social isolation, poverty, substance abuse, partner's parents had abusive relationship, personality/character disorder or mental illness.
5. H/o: Describe violent episode, what triggered it? Were objects used as weapons?
6. Injuries? Was the boyfriend remorseful afterward? H/o of previous episodes of violence or loss of temper by boyfriend.
7. What is patient's response? Has the patient been in an abusive relationship before?
8. Were the patient's parents in an abusive relationship?
9. Is boyfriend controlling, does he restrict her activities, question her excessively after she has been out, engage in verbal abuse or threats?
10. Is the violence increasing in severity? Are there children in the house?
11. Who are the biological parents? Ask about violence to the children, sexual abuse.
12. Does the patient of her partner abuse alcohol or other drugs?
13. Is money a problem? Is the boyfriend in a particularly stressful time?
14. What is the state of the patient's relationship with the boyfriend?
15. Is the boyfriend willing to seek help?
16. Counsel: Explain that the boyfriend hitting the patient is a criminal assault and an example of domestic violence.
17. DV tends to increase over time unless the victim leaves, or the abuser and couple seek therapy.
18. Very often, women don't leave their abusive partner until they are seriously hurt or killed.
19. DV between adult partners tends to be reflected in future behaviour of children who are exposed to it, and there is a risk of violence towards the children.
20. Recommend that the patient not to return to the abuser if there is risk to her safety (e.g. not the first assault, abuser not remorseful).

21. Alternatively, the patient can contact the police to obtain a restraining order on the abuser.
22. Develop a plan with the patient to seek alternate living arrangements (women's abuse shelter), list the support system (friends, other family members), contact the police (patient should be informed that, if contacted, the police will lay charges).
23. Counsel patient on how to enter into controlled, safe, contact with the abuser to discuss possible therapy for anger management and controlling behaviours, with therapy as a couple for relationship problems.
24. Refer to a social worker. Arrange follow-up.

Wound suture

Case: Suture laceration on a rubber forearm. Choose suture type. Is a tetanus booster required?

1. Suturing station: Past years have included a point for introducing yourself to the rubber forearm.
2. H/o: Occupation, mechanism of injury, environment in which injury occurred, how long since the injury?
3. Any distal loss of sensation, motor power?
4. Other injuries.
5. PMH, medications, drugs/alcohol use, smoking, allergies, ROS.
6. Choice of suture: Use non-absorbable monofilament such as 3-0 Prolene or Ethylon. Braided sutures can harbour bacteria and absorbable cause more inflammatory reaction in the skin. Given a choice between 3-0 silk (a braided non-absorbable) and chromic gut (a braided absorbable), choose silk.
7. Technique: For small wound, use interrupted stitches starting at the middle of the wound.
8. Anaesthetize with lidocaine 1% without epinephrine, cleanse and irrigate wound beforehand and drape, glove and observe sterile technique.
9. Tetanus immunization status: Dose Td 0.5 mL IM. Usual schedule of immunizations for tetanus (prepared as diphtheria-tetanus toxoid plus pertussis vaccine, i.e. DTP) is 2, 4, 6, 18 months. Td (diphtheria-tetanus toxoid) at 14-16 years, then repeat q 10 years.
10. Tetanus treatment based on the time of the last tetanus immunization.
    a. 0-5 yrs ago   none
    b. 5-10 yrs ago   boost (Td)
    c. >10 yrs ago   boost and give immunoglobulin (passive)
    d. uncertain   boost and give immunoglobulin (passive)
11. Follow-up: Warn of signs of infection.
12. Remove sutures in 7 days (5 days on face to minimize scarring, the face heals faster and is less likely to become infected due to better blood supply).
13. Recommend tylenol plain if pain is a problem.

Wrist joint examination

Case: A young alcoholic sustained a laceration to the right wrist whlile falling down. Perform a focussed P/E. Findings: Numbness on ulnar side of hand. Allen's test shows no ulnar artery refill, FDS impaired in little and ring finger. What structures are likely to be lacerated? Manage.

1. Is hand warm and pink?
2. Allen's test: Compress ulnar and radial arteries at the wrist, have patient open and close hand to remove blood, then release one side—the hand should flush pink due to blood supply from the side released.
3. Sensory: Check two-point discrimination on either side of each digit.
4. Pin-prick sensation:
5. Median nerve: Palmar side of the palm, palmar surface of the thumb, and the palmar surface and dorsal tips of the index, middle and thenar side of the ring fingers. The median nerve also innervates most muscles of the thenar eminence, and the 1st and 2nd lumbricals. The thumb is weak in abduction at 90° to the plane of the hand in median nerve dysfunction.
6. Ulnar nerve: Ulnar side of the hand.
7. Radial nerve: Dorsal surface of the thenar side of the hand.
8. Motor: Don't ask the patient to apply force against resistance as this may rupture a partially severed tendon—test active ROM only).
9. Median nerve: Thumb abduction.
10. Ulnar nerve: Finger spread against resistance.
11. Radial nerve: Wrist extension.
12. To test FDP function: Hold the MCP joints in extension and ask patient to flex DIPs.
13. To test FDS: Hold all fingers except the one you are testing in extension and ask patient to flex the remaining finger.
14. Structures lacerated: Since there is a diminished ulnar territory sensation, Allen's test shows no refill from ulnar circulation, and FDS weakness in little finger and ring finer, the following structures were included in the laceration: Ulnar nerve, ulnar artery, flexor retinaculum, ulnar two divisions of FDS.
15. Treatment: Clean and explore the wound under local anaesthesia and sterile conditions. Consult plastic surgery for microvascular repair.
16. Note: Structures superficial to the flexor retinaculum (ulnar to thenar): Ulnar nerve, ulnar artery, cutaneous branch of ulnar nerve, palmaris longus tendon, cutaneous branch of median nerve.

17. Structures deep to the flexor retinaculum (ulnar to thenar): 4 flexor digitorum superficialis tendons (FDS), median nerve, flexor carpi radialis tendon.
18. FDS flexes the MCP and PIP joints of the fingers, while flexor digitorum profundus (FDP) flexes the DIP.
19. Both the FDS and FDP can flex the entire finger, but the FDP tends to flex them all at once, while the FDS can flex fingers in isolation.

Back pain

Case: Young man with recent onset back pain and limp. Take H/o and physical.

1.   Mechanical (muscle strain/spasm or facet joint pain)
2.   Intervertebral disk bulging, herniation or rupture
3.   Spinal stenosis (narrowing) which can be caused by osteophytes, congenital narrow canal, spondylolisthesis (forward or backward slipping of one vertebra on another).
4.   Malignant tumour (e.g. in a young person), lymphoma
5.   Discitis/osteomyelitis
6.   Pyelonephritis
7.   Ankylosing spondylitis
8.   Vertebral compression fracture
9.   Malignancy
10. Malingering
11. H/o and P/E for back pain is to differentiate radiculopathy from other causes and to identify the nerve root.
12. The most common disk herniation is a posterolateral L4-5, which compresses the L5 root. The herniation will also compress the L4 root if the herniation is far lateral and the S1 root if it is more medial (central). The second most common herniation is a posterolateral L5-S1, which compresses the S1 root. (Note: In the thoracic and lumber spine, the nerve roots exit below the pedicles of the vertebra of the same number, while in the neck the nerve root exits above the pedicle of the vertebra of the same number).
13. L5 compression produces lateral calf pain, numbness of the medial dorsum of the foot (including web of great toe), and ankle dorsiflexion weakness.
14. S1 compression produces posterior calf pain, lateral foot numbness and ankle plantar flexion weakness (with decreased ankle jerk).
15. H/o: Pain, location, radiation, quality, duration, frequency and intensity.
16. Aggravating and relieving factors.
17. Onset and chronology, previous episodes. Previous investigations and treatment.
18. Pain worse on lying down and bilateral leg weakness suggests spinal stenosis or ankylosing spondylitis.
19. Spinal stenosis: Characterized by worsening of symptoms with standing and walking with relief on bending and sitting (H/o: leaning on and bending over the shopping cart for relief of pain while shopping).
20. Ankylosing spondylitis: Morning stiffness relieved by activity.
21. Mechanical back pain: pain worse in back than in buttock or leg.

22. Radiculopathy: Pain worse in buttock or leg than in back.
23. Has the patient had fever, weight loss, night sweats (signs of cancer), UTI (sign of urinary retention), joint pain, uveitis (sign of ankylosing spondylitis)?
24. Ask about effect on ADLS, functional limitations.
25. Associated numbness, weakness. Are the symptoms improving or worsening?
26. Medications, drugs and alcohol, smoking, PMH, family H/o, ROS.
27. Cauda equina syndrome: Ask about the bowel, bladder, and sexual function to reveal this rare syndrome. It consists of saddle anaesthesia (perineal numbness), lax anus, impotence, urinary retention, and bowel incontinence. These signs are due to preservation of sympathetic tone with loss of parasympathetic tone. Sympathetic tone is preserved because it is carried extra-spinally, while parasympathetic signals are carried via the inferior spine and nerve roots. Bowel contraction and penile erection are parasympathetically driven. Because these functions may not recover once lost, cauda equina syndrome due to a surgically treatable lesion is a surgical priority if the loss of function is acute.
28. Standing: gait, posture, range of motion including rotation, lateral and forward flexion, extension (pain worse on forward flexion and relief on extension suggest discogenic pain; pain worse on extension suggests facet joint pain).
29. Ankylosing spondylitis: Schober's test is positive when distance between the lumbosacral junction and a point 10 cm above (marked on the erect spine) expand by less than 5 cm on full forward flexion of the spine (patient standing; knee joint extended).
30. Scoliosis on standing (shoulder heights equal?) and also on forward flexion.
31. Inspect back for spina bifida.
32. Palpate for tenderness over sacroiliac joints.
33. Compress pelvis to elicit pain of sacroiliitis (Hallmark of ankylosing spondylitis).
34. Muscle tone.
35. Percuss at costo-vertebral angles for renal pain.
36. Can the patient walk on toes/heels.
37. Ask patient to stand on one foot at a time and push up into tiptoe for ankle plantar flexor strength (S1).
38. Sitting: Knee jerks (L2, 3, 4) with quadriceps exposed, watch contraction.
39. Ankle jerks (S1).
40. Rapidly dorsiflex each foot to test for clonus. Babinski's sign.
41. Measure calf circumference 10 cm below tibial tuberosity.
42. Power of quadriceps, hamstrings, psoas (raise knee up against resistance), ankle dorsiflexors.

43. Ask the patient to straighten both legs and compare this position to the degree of forward flexion that the patient was able to achieve on standing range of motion. Suspicion of malingering is raised if the patient claims to be unable to bend from a standing position but is able to extend the knees from a sitting position.

44. Supine: Feel for lymph nodes at neck, clavicle, axillae, and groin. Test hip extensors (patient presses leg into bed while you try to raise it).

45. Sensation at both legs: Light touch and pinprick—compare medial dorsum of foot (L5) with lateral foot (S1) and lateral calf (L5) with posterior calf (S1). Vibration and position sense in big toes.

46. Straight leg raise: Raise patient's head off bed as far as patient will allow, note angle, note whether this reproduced the patient's ipsilateral or contralateral radicular pain.

47. Bowstring test: Flex hip to 90 degrees, extend knee to the point of pain and press on the hamstring tendon which is medial. Note reproduction of pain.

48. Peripheral vascular exam: Inspect for venous stasis or arterial insufficiency ulcers, check femoral pulses and auscultate for femoral bruits, feel popliteal, dorsalis pedis, and tibialis posterior pulses.

Case: 30 yr old male with back pain and stiffness. Take H/o and perform a focussed P/E. Findings: 10 cm separation between lumbar spines while erect increases by less than 5 cm when back is flexed forward (positive Schober test), lateral flexion impaired. Give the diagnosis and 2 associated conditions

1. Back Pain H/o and P/E.
2. Predominating symptoms of stiffness are suggestive of ankylosing spondylitis. Back pain is recurring and tends to be nocturnal.
3. Morning stiffness improves over the day. May be associated with weight loss, fatigue, anaemia.
4. Focus on joint symptoms (typically large joints), uveitis (occurs in 1/3 of cases), and family H/o.
5. Diagnosis: Based on typical H/o of back pain, lumbar spine X-rays showing fusion of the SI joints or sacroiliitis and syndesmophytes (disc spaces undergoing fusion), elevated ESR and HLA-B27 tissue specific antigen.
6. Associated conditions: Inflammatory arthritis, uveitis, psoriasis, IBD, amyloidosis, radiculopathy, pericarditis, angina, conduction abnormalities.
7. Treatment: No cure. Regular therapeutic exercise to prevent deformity/disability (especially swimming and back extension exercises).
8. To control pain and stiffness—indomethacin (100 mg po OD), naproxen (250 mg po bid-tid). Surgery helpful in severe cases.

Case: 24 yr old female with LLQ abdominal pain who has an IUD. P/E Findings: signs of peritoneal irritation. Give DDx and order investigations.

1. P/E with manual and speculum exam of pelvis. Check for cervical motion tenderness (PID), pain on palpation of ovaries, mass, cervical discharge, string attached to IUD should be present at the cervix.
2. DDx: Uterine perforation by IUD, PID (PID more common with IUD), ovarian cyst with torsion or rupture, tubo-ovarian abscess, ectopic pregnancy (more common with IUD), gastroenteritis, IBD, intestinal obstruction due to volvulus or IBD.
3. Investigations: Abdominal X-rays—3 views, abdominal/pelvic U/S, CBC, lytes, BUN, Cr, INR/PTT, glucose, ?-hCG, urinalysis, stool for occult blood, cervical swabs for culture and pap smear. If OR is imminent order type and cross match for 2 units PRBCs, CXR.

Carpel Tunnel syndrome

Case: 31 yr old female with right hand numbness and weakness. Take H/o and perform focussed P/E. Give DDx, investigations, and treatment.

1.   H/o: Name, age, occupation, amount of work done with hands, description of symptoms, onset, duration, chronology, time of day, aggravating and relieving factors.
2.   Previous episodes. Ask about pain at night.
3.   Functional limitations. Difficulty turning a key or opening jars.
4.   Associated injury, neck pain, numbness or weakness in other areas, visual problems, headache, nausea.
5.   Medications, drug/alcohol use, smoking, allergies, PMH (DM, hypothyroidism, RA, pregnancy), surgical H/o, family H/o, ROS.
6.   P/E: neck exam. Check two-point discrimination at each fingertip.
7.   Median nerve territory is the palmar surface of the thumb and the palmar surface and dorsal tips of the index, middle and thenar side of the ring fingers. Sensation to the ulnar side of the hand is the ulnar nerve, and the dorsal surface of the thenar side of the hand is radial nerve innervated. The median nerve also innervates most muscles of the thenar eminence, and the 1st and 2nd lumbricals.
8.   The thumb is weak in abduction at 90° to the plane of the hand in median nerve dysfunction.
9.   Tinel's sign: Tapping the palmar surface of the wrist elicits shooting paresthesia in median distribution.
10.   Phalen's sign: Maximally flexing both wrists by pushing the dorsi of the hands together elicits median nerve distribution numbness/paraesthesia after 30-60 seconds.
11.   DDx: Carpal tunnel compression of median nerve, cervical radiculopathy, stroke, TIA, diabetic peripheral neuropathy, brachial plexus injury or tumour. Investigations: nerve conduction studies.
12.   Treatment: Modify manual work, wrist splint often worn at night, NSAIDs, local corticosteroid injections, control underlying contributors e.g. DM, hypothyroidism, arthritis, surgical decompression.

Solitary lung nodule

Case: 53 yr old female with incidental solitary lung nodule on CXR. Take H/o.

1. Ocupation, hobbies, pets esp. birds, cats, travel H/o, contact with hazardous substances (e.g. asbestos), positive TB skin test, H/o of pneumonia, smoking, alcoholism, lung symptoms: cough, sputum, SOB, hemoptysis, wheeze, orthopnea, chest wall pain.
2. Medications, drugs/alcohol, allergies, PMH, family H/o, ROS, check for malignant symptoms such as weight loss, fatigue, change of bowel habits, anorexia, night pain.
3. DDx: Granuloma (scar tissue from old pneumonia, TB granuloma, histoplasmosis, silicosis, sarcoid), tumour (benign e.g. hamartoma, primary malignant, metastatic), vascular malformation, lung abscess. Most Likely Dx: granuloma
4. Investigations: Old chest x-ray for comparison (if lesion is old and unchanging, interventions are less aggressive, calcification is also associated with benign lesions such as old granulomas).
5. CT chest with CT guided needle biopsy, sputum for cytology and acid-fast staining (TB), TB skin test, bronchoscopy with biopsy and washings if lesion seen, open biopsy or lobectomy.

Ankle injury

Case: A young man presents to the Emergency department having twisted his ankle. Manage

1. H/o of ankle strain: H/o of a plausible mechanism of injury involving significant inversion or eversion of the foot with pain and swelling.
2. Time of injury, onset of pain and swelling (may be delayed), noises heard at time of injury. Previous ankle or other injuries. Ability to walk post injury (often preserved if ligaments are not ruptured).
3. Past medical H/o, medications, allergies, family H/o).
4. P/E: Inspect for gross deformity, erythema, swelling bruising.
5. Check distal circulation, sensation, active and passive range of motion, palpate for tenderness at joints.
6. Examine the joints above and below the affected joint. Identify sites of maximal tenderness.
7. Talar drawer sign: Stabilize the tibia and pull forward on the heel, talar drawer sign is anterior movement of the talus.
8. Greater than 3 mm anterior movement may be significant, 1 cm is significant and indicates anterior talofibular ligament rupture.
9. Talar tilt: Stabilize the tibia, grasp the talus and tilt in eversion and inversion. Movement beyond the normal range (compare with the opposite side) is a positive talar tilt and indicates lateral (calcaneofibular) ligament rupture if the tilt occurs in inversion or medial (deltoid) ligament if the tilt occurs in eversion.
10. Ottawa Ankle rules:
    a. Ankle Xray is indicated only if bone tenderness over tibial or fibular malleoli or unable to bear wt. both immediately and in ER
    b. Foot Xray—bone tenderness over the base of 5th metatarsal or navicular bone or unable to bear wt. both immediately and in ER.
    c. Calcaneal views if there is pain on palpation of heel.

11. Pain in the ankle on squeezing the calf is a sign of ankle fracture.
12. Treatment for ankle sprain: Rest, use crutches, avoid weight bearing. Ice for 20 min qid for 2-3 days. Compression with tensor bandage or tape. Elevate.
13. Rehabilitation: start active range of motion exercises 2 days post injury, may weight bear after pain and swelling have subsided.

14. Full ligament healing may take 6 weeks in severe injury or more if re-injury occurs.
15. Complete ligament rupture with joint instability (positive talar drawer sign or talar tilt) should be evaluated by Orthopedics.

Disc herniation

Case: 70 yr old male with neck pain and left arm weakness. Perform a focussed P/E. Findings: Decreased sensation over left index and middle finger, mild wrist extensor and triceps weakness. Describe a cervical spine film of the patient's neck (shows narrowing of C6-C7 disc space). Give diagnosis and treatment.

1. Musculoskeletal, discogenic, stenotic, malignant, or brainstem infarct.
2. Take vitals.
3. Examine cranial nerves: Pupillary reflexes, extra-ocular movements, visual fields, facial muscles (raise eyebrows, show teeth, protrude tongue), facial sensation, gag, Horner's syndrome, sternomastoid and trapezius muscle power.
4. Cerebellar testing: Finger-nose, heel-shin, dysdiadocokinesis, gait, Rhomberg test, pronator drift.
5. Neck: Inspect for lesions, asymmetry, muscle wasting of sternomastoids, palpate for nodes, masses, palpate dorsal vertebral spines and range of motion.
6. Shoulders, arms, hands: inspect for symmetry, wasting, fasciculations, skin lesions.
7. Power: Test deltoids (C5), biceps (C6), triceps and wrist extension (C7), hand intrinsics (C8). Note that each muscle group actually has mixed nerve root innervation, i.e. deltoids and biceps (C5, 6), triceps (C6, 7, 8), wrist extension (C6, 7), hand intrinsics (C8, T1).
8. Sensation: Check pinprick, vibration, light touch over the shoulder (C5), thumb (C6), index and middle finger (C7), ring and little finger (C8).
9. Deep tendon reflexes: Biceps, triceps, brachioradialis. Hoffman's sign (the Babinski of the upper limb: flick relaxed index finger dorsally, thumb abducts in a +ive test).
10. Tone/Rigidity: check for increased tone by rapid supination or extension of elbow.
11. C-spine X-rays:
    a. Lateral view: An adequate lateral shows the top of the T1 vertebra. Look for alignment of the anterior and posterior margins of vertebral bodies as well as spinous processes. Spinous processes may have abnormal separation in injury. The maximal normal distance between the posterior aspect of the anterior arch of C1 and the dens is 3 mm in adults and 5 mm in children (more in RA). Look for regularity of disk space height, gas in the disk space (suggests degeneration), osteophytes, pre-vertebral swelling greater than one third of the vertebral body width (7 mm from C1-4, 22 mm from C5-7).

Hangman's fracture: coronal plane fracture through the base of both pedicles of C2, caused by hyperextension injury, separates the posterior elements of C2 from its body.

b. *AP view*: Check the alignment of processes and vertebral bodies, distance between spinous processes should be regular. Erosion of a pedicle is seen as "winking owl sign" where the pedicles are the eyes and the spinous process, the beak.

c. *Odontoid view*: Misalignment of outline of the cortex of the bone indicates odontoid fracture. Odontoid fracture type I: tip, type II: base, type III: through body of C2.

12. Diagnosis: A narrowed C6, 7 disk space suggests disk degeneration at that level. C6, 7 disk herniation impinges on the C7 nerve root and produce C6, 7 nerve root dysfunction on sensory and motor exam.

13. Treatment: Most patients respond to conservative therapy: Soft collar, NSAID, acetaminophen.

14. Refer to neurosurgery for myelogram, CT neck and CT myelogram. May require decompressive laminectomy or anterior discectomy with bone graft fusion.

Section 10

Professional and Ethical issues

Breaking bad news

Breaking bad news is one of the most difficult tasks a physician or other member of the health care team has to do. The way it is done may change the nature of the relationship permanently—strengthen it, undermine it, damage it irreparably or even leading to litigation.

1. Get the setting right: Use basic communication and facilitation skills, ensure privacy, get the body language right and make eye contact.
2. Find out what the patient knows already: Ask the patient what s/he already knows or suspect, what were you told? What have you figured out?
    Listen to the way in which the patient describes the situation, noting the vocabulary used and the level of comprehension as well as denial.
3. Find out what the patient wants: Obtain a clear invitation to share information if this is what s/he wants to know. The results of your tests have come out. Some of the results are little complex to explain. Do you want to know all about it? Are you a kind of person who wants to know every detail of the result? Do you want to have some one with you if some of the results are going to be very bad? What are your expectations about the results?
4. Give information: Start at the level of patient's comprehension and use the same vocabulary, cultural sensitivity. Give information in small chunks and in simple language, and checking regularly to see whether the content is understood. If the patient cries, offer napkins and keep silent for some time.
5. Responding to the patient's feelings: Acknowledge all reactions. Use the empathic response technique. Identify emotion and cause of emotion, and respond to show the patient that this connection has been made. Deal with crying (napkin), anger and other strong emotions. Say that you understood the feelings.
6. Offer him that you can talk to his partner provided s/he give him consent. In case of communicable STDs even if he denies consent, tell him that his partner will be informed by the public health authorities. Now the patient might become angry. Tell the patient that the public health authorities will not tell the partner that s/he is infected. They will only tell him/her that the person with whom s/he had sexual relationship is having the test positive. It is up to him/her to assume who that would be.
7. Closing: Summarize the major areas discussed. Ask the patient whether there are other important questions or issues that he or she wishes to discuss now. Make a clear contract for the next meeting.

Barriers and challenges: Denying the illness, use of professional language, fear of diminishing the patient's hope, repressing your feelings, and vanishing.

Decision to forgo

Case 1: Mrs. X is a 25 years old woman requesting the removal of her respirator. She has been diagnosed with chronic Gillen-Barre syndrome. There is no hope for her to recover. Talk to her.

Case 2: Ms. X is asking for a DNR order to be written on her mother's chart without her mother's knowledge. Her mother has chronic congestive heart failure and her health has deteriorated over the past 5 years. Talk to the patient's daughter.

Case 3: Mrs. X wants to speak with the emergency physician about her mother (Mrs. Y) who is unconscious and bleeding as a result of a head-on collision. Both are both Jehovah's Witnesses. Talk to Mrs. X.

Case 4: Mrs. X wants information about her husband Y's condition. Y has suffered a cerebral aneurysm 4 days ago. He has been declared "brain dead" by a neurologist and a neurosurgeon. Please tell the wife about his status and what you propose to do.

Dealing with the situation

1.   Ask the reason to stop/refuse treatment.
2.   Take a brief mental status exam/mood/psychotic screen.
3.   Discuss with other family members if necessary
4.   Establish medical competence: Make sure that the patient understands the disease, the treatment options, and the consequences of no treatment.
5.   The patient has the right to refuse treatment.
6.   Offer counseling and social support.
7.   Discuss the patient's competence to take decisions on life-support measures.
8.   In future admissions: discuss the role of advance directives, keeping substitute decision-makers and living will.
9.   Discuss the right to change his/her decision.
10.   Make arrangements so other staff members will know about it.

If the patient is in an unconscious vegetative state:

1.   Discuss with the family the reason to stop treatment.
2.   Patient's opinion/whishes/living will towards prolonging life.
3.   Offer support and counseling to the family (when condition is terminal).

If Jehovah's witness's "no transfusion" is the issue: Explain the seriousness of the condition: the patient will die w/o the blood transfusion.
1.   Is the family member a substitute decision-maker?
2.   Are there other substitute decision-makers?

3. Does the patient have a card? Date of issue? Still an active member?
4. Previous wishes expressed by the patient with regard to transfusions?
5. Would the patient choose to die because of not getting blood?

Telling the truth

Case 1: X is a 20 years old man university student. He appears well, but is requesting a note saying that he is too sick to write the exam tomorrow. Interview him.
Case 2: You are about to see Mrs. X, the wife of a man who has been diagnosed as having pancreatic cancer. The tumor is inoperable and he is terminally ill. She is requesting not to tell him the truth regarding is condition. Interview her.
Case 3: Mr. X is a 62 years old man who comes to your office for results of neuropsychological and neurological testing. According to neurologist, Mr. X has a clinical presentation of Alzheimer's disease. Interview him and address his questions.

Dealing with the station:

1. Investigate why the family does not want the patient knows about the diagnosis.
2. Investigate the patient's family situation, is cancer the problem word?
3. Ask about previous statement from the patient, living will, psychiatric H/o.
4. Be gentle. But establish that you cannot lie to the patient. S/he has the right to know about the Dx, this is based in the principle of trust between the doctor and his/her patient. If the patient find out, he/she will think that there is a plot against him/her affecting the doctor-patient relationship. Argue that nowadays the patients are very intelligent and get information from the internet confronting physician very often.
5. Tell the family that you will be very gentle with the patient. You can deal with the consequences.
6. Tell the family that by knowing the truth, the patient will be able to make decisions in terms of how far to go with treatments and procedures. e.g.DNR.
7. Refuse to promise not to tell the truth although you will not volunteer the diagnosis if the patient does not want to know.
8. Finally offer support, counseling, psychological assessment.
9. Thus disclosing the truth will promote patient well being, furthers patient's choices in life, shows respect for the person and reduce physician's liability.

Battered woman

Case 1: Mrs. X is a 30 years old woman who comes to see you because of irregularities in her periods. Interview her.
Case 2: Mr. X is a 35 years old woman who comes to see you requesting tranquilizers because she has been on edge, under a lot of stress and has trouble sleeping. Interview.
Case 3: Mrs. X is a 29 years old woman who is 28 weeks of pregnancy. She comes to see you for a regular heck up and you notice a cast on her right arm. Interview her.

Dealing with the situation:

1. Take a brief H/o about the present complaints......get into the topic carefully.
2. Assess the risk factors: Single mother, family H/o of abuse, alcohol, drug abuse, police involvement, small children.
3. Get into psychosocial H/o: Pay attention to the patient's gestures, reaction, silences and body language.
4. Be honest and direct: Ae suffering from any kind of abuse? Physical abuse?
5. Get into the incident in details: When was the last time, since when, how, how many times, children abuse too? Police involved? Weapons? Did he threaten to kill you? Hospitalizations? Broken bones? Alcohol/drugs involved?
6. Who knows about it? Family, neighbor's friends. Any support at all?
7. Patient's feelings: mood, suicidal, homicidal?
8. Explain that this is a crime in Canada. Nobody has the right to treat you like this. Express concerns regarding the patient and the children's safety. Explain that violence has a negative impact on children.
9. Start developing a plan.
10. Ask the patient if she wants to go back home? Remember that is her decision.
11. Offer referral to social worker, community resources, and shelters.
12. Also, offer help for the partner, remember that most of this woman do not want to leave their partner ("He is a good guy").

Autopsy/Organ donation

Case 1: You are going to see Mrs. X. Her husband was brought by paramedics 2 hrs ago with an acute MI and despite the work of the ER team, he die of complications. Talk to her and request an autopsy.

Case 2: Mr. X is a 30 years old man who suffered a MVA a week ago. He was declared "brain dead" by a Neurologist and a neurosurgeon. You are going to talk to Mrs. X (the wife) and talk about organ donation.

Case 3: A 47 years old female well-controlled IDDM was brought by paramedics to ER. The patient was already dead on the arrival to the hospital. You are the physician on duty who received the patient. You are going to talk to Mr. X (the patient's husband) about it. Talk to him and try to find out what happened.

Approaching the cases:
1. You may have to deal with "breaking bad news", so be gentle.... And take your time.
2. Say that you sorry for the loss. And keep silence for a few seconds......Repeat it.......Offer napkin.
3. Case 1: Explain that in spite of the effort of the medical team Mr. X passed away due to his serious condition. When the autopsy issue comes, explain that is not a disfiguring procedure to the body, that does not take long, it will not interfere with the funeral, and that she can refuse. Offer that she can see the body, that some tubes may be coming out of it and also offer help and support contacting family.
4. Case 2: Point out that this is a difficult situation. There is no hope that her husband will recuperate. Bring up the issue of "Organ Donation". Ask if he ever discussed it before? Any paper signed? Go slowly into the topic. Explain that he is a good candidate for donation because he is young and healthy. She may take some time to think and talk to the rest of the family, but unfortunately, the procedure should be done under certain conditions and we can not wait days. Talk about the benefits of helping people waiting for transplant, comment about the procedure, the team, and by protocol. She won't know who is going to receive the organs. Emphasize that she is not under the obligation to agree and any moral, religious or personal believes will be respected.
5. Case 3: Try to find out about what happened the night she was found unconscious. Who gave her insulin, how familiar the husband was with the treatments and side effects of DM and insulin therapy. Ask about the previous day, symptoms of depression, complications of DM, previous hospitalizations, how well the patient was taking care of her disease.

6. When the time comes, bring up the autopsy issue and see their reaction. It will help to understand what really happened. Explain that when a patient arrives in the hospital in coma and die within the first 24 hrs, the Coroner takes part in the case and the autopsy is obligatory.

7. Offer help.

Drug Seeker

Case 1: Ms.X is a 29 years old nurse who comes to your office for the first time because of bad headaches. She is requesting a prescription for Percoset. Talk to her.

1. Start taking a brief H/o about the patient…..Remember that is the first time that you see him/her.
2. Find out who prescribed narcotics before, for how long, H/o of headaches, change of physicians, cities, investigate social H/o, substance abuse.
3. Establish how many milligrams is he taking (probably a lot) and point out your concerns regarding his taking a high doses of narcotics for headaches.
4. Ask about withdrawal symptoms, and say that you think that he/she is hooked to the narcotics. Address this as a problem.
5. Explain that actually by prescribing narcotics you may worsen the pain (vicious cycle). Recognize her/his dependence to medication and offer help.
6. Suggest referral to clinics or rehabilitation centers to start treatment.
7. Deal with the patient's anger. It seems that you are becoming angry. Can you tell me the reason?
8. (Be firm and convinced about what you should do). We do not prescribe narcotics during the first visit. If you go to another clinic, they will tell you the same.
9. Address the pain and offer him/her substitute painkiller (e.g. Keterolac) to alleviate symptoms.
10. Offer follow up.

Case 2: 25 yr old man who consumed an entire prescription of Florinal in 4 days wishes to refill a prescription for tension headache. Manage.

1. Description of headache pain, location, quality, intensity, duration, onset including time of day (morning headache associated with raised intracranial pressure).
2. Previous episodes, aggravating factors, relieving factors (e.g. coughing and bending worsen headache in raised ICP, and chocolate, cheeses can trigger migraines).
3. Associated symptoms (aura, nausea, vomiting, photophobia, phonophobia, nuchal rigidity, weakness, numbness, and visual disturbances).
4. Past medical H/o, current medications, allergies.
5. Family H/o, substance abuse, smoking, mood, stress, anxiety.
6. ROS.

7. Suggest to the examiner that you would perform a brief neurological screening exam.

8. Explain that Florinal is mixture of barbiturate and ASA which is used only for the relief of occasional tension headaches.

9. It is habit—forming, can cause withdrawal syndrome consisting of agitation, delirium and seizures, and has sedative effects.

10. Since patient consumed full prescription in 4 days, it suggests overuse due to dependence.

11. He may have analgesic headache syndrome where inappropriate analgesic use cause headaches.

12. Suggest a drug holiday with weaning from caffeine and alcohol.

13. Advise proper sleep hygiene, diet, exercise and stress management.

14. Chronic headache may also be a symptom of depression or anxiety.

15. Offer follow up.

HIV and Ethics

Case 1: Mrs. X is a 31 year old nurse who works in the hospital. About 1 hour ago she suffered a needle stick injury in her hand when trying to transfuse a patient. She is now coming to talk to you regarding HIV risks. Interview her.

Case 2: Ms. X is a 29 year old woman who comes to talk to you regarding the HIV test. Her boyfriend was recently hospitalized because of PCP. Counsel.

Case 3: Mr. X is a 35 year old man who comes asking for the HIV test. He works as an airline pilot and wants to talk to you regarding the test. Interview him.

Case 4: Mr. X is a 28 year old man who is coming to receive the results of an ELISA. The test is (+). Talk to him.

Case 1

1. When did it happen?
2. Ask about significant exposure to blood/body fluids.
3. Were you wearing gloves? Fresh blood on the needle?
4. Did the wound bleed? How deep was the injury?
5. Did you wash the wound with water/soap/iodine?
6. Ask about the patient.
7. Why was the patient in the hospital? HIV status? Hepatitis status?
8. Sexual H/o in detail: partner/s, HIV status, STDs, safe sex, mode of intercourse.
9. Risk factors for blood transmitted diseases?
10. Did you ask him/her about doing an HIV test?
11. Ask about the nurse's vaccination status (Hepatitis, Tetanus).
12. Tell about notifying the "occupational health office"
13. Assess risk behavior: Previous accidents, how long in this profession, drugs, tattoos, transfusions, artificial insemination.

Counseling for case 1, 2 and 3:

1. Here is when you are going to give information to the patient and also answer questions. So be prepared.
2. Risk in heterosexual couple of getting HIV in 1 year of unprotected sex: 16-20%
3. Risk if sharing needles: 99.5%
4. Tell that you need informed consent for ELISA. Explain that it detects antibodies. If negative should be repeated in 6 weeks, 12 weeks, 6 months (window period).
5. The results will arrive after 2-4 wks. The test can be sent with his/her name/or anonymous.

6. Explain the difference between being HIV and having AIDS.
7. Explain that it is better to come with someone to receive the results (the result is given only in person).
8. Offer counseling, support, reading material, contact partners if (+). Talk a little bit about treatment and that this is a chronic infection.
9. In the mean time, until results are available, patient should practice safe sex (condoms).

Case 4:
1. You are going to break a bad news. Be prepared and gentle.
2. Ask if the first time that the patient has the HIV test done.
3. The patient will be eager to know the results. Calm him down. Don't give the results straight away.
4. First ask the patient how much he wants to know about the results? Everything?
5. Are you a kind of person who wants to know everything?
6. Do you want to have someone with you when I explain the complex results? What are your expectations about the results today?
7. I am afraid I have bad news.......The test came back (+)..... Patient is going to cry. I am sorry..............wait and repeat........I am sorry..........Keep silence for 15 sec.
8. Say that you understand that this is very shocking.
9. Ask if the patient was expecting the positive results?
10. This is not the end of your life. Take your time to accept it.
11. Talk about the variability in the prognosis.
12. Explain the difference of HIV positive state and AIDS.
13. Outline some studies that you are going to do, F/Us, therapies and prophylaxis. Outline changes in lifestyle (good nutrition, exercise, decrease stress).
14. Never: Share razors, tooth brush, give blood, organ donation.
15. Safe sex: Using condoms. If in a relationship, encourage to discuss and bring the partner for testing. Contact previous partners.
16. Offer your help to talk to the partner/s.
17. If he does not want his wife know about it, tell him that 'by law' the blood results are going to be reported to public health department. Some one from the public health department will contact his partner. They are not going to say that you are HIV+. They will only say that someone with whom she had sex is suffering from HIV+. It is up your partner to assume who that can be.
18. Finally, offer psychological support, flyers, information, group supports and ask the patient to call you any time.

Case 1. Offer AZT prophylaxis and hepatitis prophylaxis if applies.
Case 3. Encourage the patient to bring his wife for testing. Support the idea of discussion about the disease.

Substance abuse and ethics

Case 1: Mr. X is a 38 year old man who comes to see you because of enlargement of the breast, (he was embarrassed to tell the nurse). Talk to him.
Case 2: Mrs. X is a mother of a 16 year old boy. She is coming to talk to you because she says she found "marihuana" in his son's pocket a few days ago. Talk to her.
Case 3: Mr. X is a 29 year old man who presented in ER last week with an episode of epistaxis. After treatment, he was referred to the family physician for F/U. The ER note says that he is using cocaine currently. You are going to talk to him for the first time.

1. Start your interview with an open question.
2. Ask about any physical complaints/withdrawal symptoms? (Be aware that in case 1 the patient may be denying his drinking problems. So be careful how you approach it).
3. Take a good social H/o: Occupation, unemployed at the moment?
4. Trouble with the police? Jail? Financial situation? Family? Relationships? Marital status?
5. *For drugs:* Since when, how often, how much, what kind, what route, complications.
   For alcohol: CAGE questionnaire. Good screening test. How much does the patient drink/day/week.
6. Drinking and driving? Why do you think you need to drink?
   Can you control it? What triggers your drinking?
   Besides drinking, also drugs? smoking?
   Investigate the behavior when drinking.
7. Toxicity: Liver, Cushing's features, testicular atrophy.

Case 2:
1. Take a good social H/o, school performance, friends, and girl friend. Problems with police, stealing money from parents, others?
2. Change in behavior? depression? family relationship?
3. Brothers/sisters? What is he doing in the free time?
4. Places he goes? Alcohol, smoking, previous drug abuse?
5. Who gives him money?
6. Take a brief PMH, medications, and hospitalizations.
7. Start your counseling: For drugs: recognize the abuse/dependence: offer help, centers for rehabilitation, detoxification therapy, group support, family involvement, community support.

8. <u>For alcohol:</u> *AA* program, family involvement, explain the dangers of drinking. Assess the risk of suicide and violence psychiatric diseases, chronic pain.
9. Address the possibility of relapsing. It is not going to be easy. Make continuous F/Us.
10. Encourage to bring the patient to the office next time and involve the family and school staff.

Confidentiality

Case 1: Mrs. X is asking for information about her daughter Linda's visits to your office. Mrs. X suspects that Linda is sexually active and is taking the pill. Both are your patients. Talk to Mrs. X.

Case 2: Mr. X requests result of HIV test which is +ive. Mr. X does not want his wife to know his HIV status. Talk to him

Case 3: Ms. X is a 15 years old woman who is requesting BCP and an HIV test because she had unprotected sex. During the interview she reveals that she missed her last period. The pregnancy test comes back (+). She requests an abortion. She asks you not to tell her parents. Talk to her. Council regarding the BCP and HIV.

1. Does she understand the risks of the abortion?
2. Encourage to her the parents.
3. HEEADSS (Home, Education, Eating, Activities, Drugs, Sex, Suicide)
4. Good relationship with parents.
5. Was she under the effect of alcohol?
6. Are they in good health?
7. Crampy, pains, infection.
8. Affecting infertility.
9. What is the purpose of today's visit?
10. Options for pregnancy.
11. Only the woman has the right for the baby.
12. Gynecological exam and a pap smear.
13. Confidentiality provides a foundation for trust in therapeutic relationship.
14. Physician should disclose information to a third party only with the consent of the patient or his/her authorized representatives or when required by law.

Obtaining consent

Case 1: Mr. X is a 66 years old man who presented 2 episodes of amaurosis fugax in the last month. The carotid angiogram was done and shows 90% obstruction at the right side. You are going to see him and report the results. Try to obtain consent for endarterectomy and address his questions.

Case 2: Mr. X is a 76 years old man who suffers from severe Alzheimer's disease. He resides in a nursing home and is unable to take care of himself. He presents with 48hrs of fever, cough, SOB and is sent to the hospital for treatment of suspected pneumonia. The nursing home has already notified Mr. X's wife, who is now on her way to the hospital. Talk to her.

Consent is the authorization of a medical intervention by individual patients. Proper consent has 3 components.
1. Disclosure: Physician should provide relevant information and patient should comprehend this information
2. Capacity: Patient should understand the relevant information and should be able to appreciate the consequence of her/his decision.
3. Free decision: Patient's right to come to a decision freely, without force or manipulation.

An informed consent should include:
1. Clearly explain nature of the procedure/intervention: Use clear language.
2. Options to the proposed treatment: Delay v/s go for it e.g. you are already receiving the full doses of medication and still you have symptoms.
3. Treatment benefits v/s those without treatment.
4. Discuss potential benefits of Rx: e.g. decrease the chances future strokes
5. Discuss potential harms.
6. Discuss benefits and risks of alternative treatments.
7. Patient's situation: how much information you can disclose to this patient, education, language, family support, job, financial situation, special plans, culture-religion, worries.
8. What functions the patient will sacrifice: If you get any post-intervention disability, is anything in your life that would be ruined? In case of post procedure disability how protected (Insurance) is this patient? Invite the family in the discussion.
9. Answer the patient's questions: make sure that the patient understood. Ask to explain in his/her language.

10. Consent may be explicit (oral/written) or implied (Indication of the willingness to undergo a certain procedure or treatment by his/her own behavior. e.g. Showing a hand for an injection. Signed consent form documents can not replace the consent process.

Assessment of capacity

Case 1: Mrs. X is a 65 years old woman who was diagnosed with non-surgical lung cancer stage III with metastasis to C1-C2. She was offered chemotherapy and radiation, but she refused. The patient has 6 months of life without treatment. Talk to her and answer her questions.

Case 2: Mr. X is a 70 years old diabetic patient who is suffering from gangrene in his right foot and lower leg. The patient originally agrees to amputation of the leg, but on the morning scheduled for the operation he refuses to give consent. Talk to him and address his questions.

Case 3: Mrs. X is a 65 years old woman who was diagnosed with colon cancer stage Ia few days ago. Although the surgeon has explained to her that a surgery will be curative, she refuses to consent to the surgery. Talk to her and answer her questions.

A typical capacity assessment consists of the following questions and is scored as follows

1.   What problems are you having now?
2.   What is the treatment for this problem?
3.   Are there any other treatment available?
4.   Can you refuse the treatment?
5.   What could happen if you have the treatment?
6.   What could happen if you don't have treatment?
7a. Test for depression (Why don't you want to have surgery?) .
7b. Test whether the person's decision is affected by delusions/psychosis

a.   Suggested scoring fall into 3 types—Yes, unsure and no.
b.   Indicate your score for each domain with a checkmark.
c.   The final result falls into the following: Definitely capable, probably capable, definitely incapable, and probably incapable.
d.   Never base a finding of incapacity solely on your interpretation of depression, delution or psychosis. If you are sure that the decision is based on a delusion or depression, always get a second independent assessment.
e.   The following does not warrant incapacity in a patient—Old age, illiteracy, physical inability to communicate, different religious background, unusual believes, psychiatric illness, refusal of treatment.

Violent behavior

Case: 30 yr old male, married with 2 children. Brought in by police for violent and dangerous behaviour. Take H/o. Would you admit this patient? What are the criteria for a Form 1?

1. Attempt to determine whether patient is sad (depressed), bad (antisocial, reaction to stressful or frustrating events, poor anger management), or mad (mania, schizophrenia).
2. Is the episode related to drugs of abuse or organic (brain tumour, metabolic disturbance)?
3. Take H/o for depression, mania, and schizophrenia with mental status exam and MMSE.
4. Criteria for admission: Patient requires observation or medication in a controlled, safe setting for diagnosis, patient appears to be a danger to himself or others, environment at home unsuitable for the patient at this time, and patient requires medical work-up for organic causes, patient in need of detoxification.
5. Criteria for a Form 1 (Involuntary hospitalization in Canada): Forcible admission for assessment without right to appeal for a maximum duration of 72 hours can be administered by any licensed physician who has seen the patient within a week.
6. Both the following criteria must be met: 1. Patient appears to be a danger to himself or others, 2. Patient appears to be currently suffering from a mental illness.

Sexual assault manage

1. Assess mental status.
2. Remove clothes and place in a plastic bag/document abrasions/bruises etc.
3. Pelvic exam and specimen collection—pubic hair combings
4. Speculum lubricate with water only/pap smear.
5. Oral cervical rectal culture for gonorrhoea and chlamydia/posterior fornix secretions.
6. Finger nail scrapings/saliva sample from victim.
7. VDRL repeat 3 months if negative/serum beta HCG.
8. Involve local or regional sexual assault team.
9. Tetanus prophylaxis.
10. Is assumed positive for gonorrhoea and Chlamydia—azithromycin 1gm PO one dose + cefixime 400 mg PO one dose.
11. Start prophylaxis for hepatitis B and HIV.
12. Pregnancy prophylaxis—Ovral 2tabs STAT +2 tabs 12 hours (within 72 hrs post coital) with Gravol 50mgm/change and shower after examination.

Ethical Issues

1. Euthanasia—one person ending another person's suffering. Physician-assisted suicide—Act of intentionally killing oneself with the assistance of a physician. Both are punishable offences under Canadian criminal law.

2. Maternal-Fetal conflict of rights—Canadian law upholds a woman's right to life and has not recognized the fetal rights. If a woman is competent and refuses medical treatment her decision must be respected even if fetus will suffer as a result. Fetus has no legal rights until it is born alive. A physician must respect the right of a competent pregnant woman patient to accept or reject any medical care recommended.

3. Induced abortion: Should not be used as an alternative to contraception. Counseling on contraception must be readily available—immediately. No delay in provision of abortion services. Physicians should not be compelled or discriminated or punished. Induced abortion should be uniformly available to all women in Canada and health care insurance should cover the costs.

4. Consent: Capable patients can refuse Rx. This decision must be respected even if it leads to serious harm or death. An incapable patient can be treated unless they refused treatment earlier when they were capable of self-determination.

5. Confidentiality: Can be disclosed when public interest overrides the patient right to confidentiality.

6. Sexual conduct with patients, even when consent by the patient is a serious matter that will lead to criminal, civil and disciplinary action.

7. Patient can change his/her mind at any time. Ask the patient to let you know.

8. Are there any family members whom Mr. X would like to involve in the decision making process.

9. Inform about all treatment outcomes including failures.

10. Manage all emergency cases when you don't know the patient's wishes/consent.

11. Capacity assessment can be combined with MMSE.

12. Where a patient cannot express his/her wishes, patient's previously expressed wishes regarding therapy should be followed.

13. Patient with drug overdose was brought in coma. First intubate her and manage. If later on you find out that s/he has a will stating no intubation, and then seek court authorization for removing her from ventilator. If any uncertainty exists, regarding patient's commitment to a previous wish, then life-sustaining treatment is given until things are clarified. May even need to seek court authorization. Sometimes the bystander will tell you that patient has a will not to intubate. If you don't see it and cannot make a clear decision about it, intubate until you clarify it. Later get court authorization to get it removed. Also you are safe to make sure that she was competent enough at the time of writing the advanced directive.

14. If patient wants your help to make an advanced directive show him an example of a living will. Help him to update it. Direct him to free legal advice centers. If the patient has any doubts about the legal validity refer to a lawyer. Also tell that if the situation changes s/he can update the advanced directive.

15. Terminally ill patient is being transferred to palliative care. Patient asks for full treatment. Educate the patient. Tell him that by treating him you will be doing more harm than good (non-malafacience).

16. In difficult situations of managing a patient inform hospital ethical committee.

17. 65 year old with MI in ICU wants to go home. Test for competency and MMSE. If there are no problems tell him what might happen and then send him home. Thus a physician is supposed to honor a competent patient's refusal of life-sustaining care.

18. A patient with carcinoma colon says that he has only some gastritis. Hospital records show that he has carcinoma colon. This is a defense mechanism. They have the right to maintain it. Ask whether the patient wants to know more about his health problem. If he says no then don't tell him anything.

19. 80 year old with dementia stopped eating. Look at his will. If not mentioned then talk to his substitute decision maker.

20. DNR orders—Give all other care for the patient. In difficult cases inform the hospital ethical committee.

21. A victim of spousal abuse is in ER now. She tells you not to tell about it to anyone. You should not tell it to any one. But you can tell the patient to reveal it to the ER staff. Also tell the patient this will not be reported to the police unless she gives consent.

22. Information received about a patient from the relatives need to be verified. First encourage the relatives to discuss it with the patient.

23. Husband with syphilis is asking you to treat the wife without telling her about him. First encourage the husband to tell her. Use it as an opportunity to discuss their marriage. If he cannot tell her, then ask for his consent to you so that you will be able to tell her. If that is also not possible tell her that public authorities will be contacting her. Assure him that they will not tell her that he is suffering from the illness. It will be up to her to assume who that will be.

24. Mandatory disclosure of the medical condition to the public health authorities should be done in case of communicable diseases, childe abuse andneglect, vulnerable adult, driving/flying safety and dangerous patients. Physician sexual misconduct should be reported to the college of physicians and surgeons of the concerned province. No need to report about physician that you think is unfit to practice.

25. If employer/insurance company asks for health status-need consent from the patient.

26. Chicken pox in pregnancy. Tell he patient about the limb abnormalities and cortical atrophy associated. Discuss the option for a therapeutic abortion.

27. An infant rolls down the exam table. Tell the parent s about it and get the child examined by another physician.

28. Old patient with pancreatic cancer. Don't know English. Family members don't want to disclose the diagnosis to her. Don't use the family members as

interpreters. Patient should be offered a chance to tell the doctor how much s/he wants to know.

29. If a daughter who living far away from the mother brought the mother to ER. Ask if there is anyone else at home who is close to her and who knows better about the patient wishes and will be able to decide the treatment in the best interests of the mother.

30. You are planning for a surgery with the patient. While getting informed consent explain the exact nature, alternatives, prognosis with and without surgery, risks and benefits of surgery, any serious effects even if unlikely, answer all the patient's questions. If patient has mental incapacity take consent from the substitute decision maker.

31. AIDS related dementia—not capable of decisions. The decreasing order of preference of substitute decision makers
    Court appointed guardian—Power of attorney—Consent capacity and review board—Partner (any one who has lived together for more than 1 year)—son/daughter/parent—noncustodial parent—sibling—any other relative.
    Public guardian and trustee (for an orphan)—Call them for all decisions.

32. You are doing a gastroscopy and patient tells you to stop. Then stop it

33. Incompetent patient refuse admission for a seriously ill disease—Admit him.

34. It is the duty of the patient to see that the benefits of a proposed Rx outweigh the risks and explain it to the patient. Then it is up to the patient to agree with you and take the risks of the intervention.

35. Report all child abuses to Children's Aid Society (CAS).

36. If a child in not capable of making decisions on his/her own, and if parents deny a life saving procedure, you should carry out all the protocols. But if the child is capable of understanding the consequences and benefits of doing the procedure and then denies the procedure then you need not do it. What should be the age of the patient? There is no age limit for this.

37. A brain dead patient in ICU. Family members insist not to do apnea test (test by stopping the mechanical ventilator). Explain to the patient that a

brain dead patient is considered as dead patient. It was confirmed by a neurologist and a neurosurgeon. Patient should be given chances to be with the patient before, during and after such discontinuation. Family members have no choice in this decision. Discuss about organ donation if the driver's license of the patient gives agreement.

38. While considering allocation of medical facilities to treatment do not consider the patients' income, patient's voluntary contribution to the illness, past use of the medical resources etc.

39. Can a psychiatric patient give a valid consent? Yes. If s/he is capable. A formal test of competence need to be done. If s/he has delusion of reference with someone outside the hospital, yes proceed with surgery.

40. If a patient is dangerous to him/herself—involuntary treatment can be given in ER. Then further treatment can be given under the authorization from a substitute decision maker.

41. If a patient wants to stop all life sustaining treatment. Before stopping
    a. Establish diagnosis
    b. Explore all options
    c. Ensure the maximum physical comfort of the patient
    d. Ensure that the patient is mentally capable
    e. Not influenced by others
    f. Involve significant others if s/he wish
    g. Consult specialist if needed
    h. Final decision with patient, significant others and the treatment team
    i. Ensure that the treatment is defensible and reasonable

42. ER has no room to keep. Offer treatment in ER. Tell the patient. Contact the hospital administrator to bring additional staff.

43. Care at end of life—Manage pain. If already incubated discuss with the patient and take advanced directives regarding future intubations. Support him/her and family.

44. Placebo controlled study in a medical condition—Placebo can be given only when there is no real and proved medication for the illness and the trail medication is equivocal to the placebo.

45. Physicians are supposed to discuss the results of the tests as it comes. Should not wait until the confirmatory test results come (especially it takes more time).

46. If the children are the substitute decision makers eligible from the list and if all 5 of them differ in opinion—refer to Consent capacity and review board (CCRB) or court.

47. A daughter is the substitute decision maker and is in doubt about the decision. How to help. Ask her whether she knows what her mother would want if the situation deteriorates further.

48. Alleviate the pain of a terminally ill patient. The decisions taken by the patient should not be influenced by the pain.

49. Husband is HIV positive. Wife is pregnant and refuses HIV test. Respect the patient's wishes even if the fetus is going to get affected. Fetus gets a choice only after delivery. Until then mother's choice will be completely respected. e.g. 2. Fetal hypoxia—need CS—Mother refuses—respect the decision.

50. Children's decisions—educate them with a psychologist or psychotherapist if needed.

51. Antibiotics to schizophrenia patient—if s/he knows the consequences/side effects like rash, diarrhea etc. prescribe it.

52. Carotid enderarterectomy—risk of stroke within 6 months is higher with surgery than medical treatment. Tell this to patient.

53. Patient wants surgery. But don't want to know the side effects. What to do? Arrange with the patient to talk to family members. Discuss and go for surgery.

54. Confidentiality: Can be disclosed when public interest overrides the patient right to confidentiality.

55. Sexual conduct with patients, even with patient consent is a serous matter that will lead to criminal, civil and disciplinary action.

56. Euthanasia—one person ending another person's suffering. Physician-assisted suicide—Act of intentionally killing oneself with the assistance of a physician. Both are punishable offences under Canadian Criminal law.

57. Maternal-Fetal conflict of rights—Canadian law upholds a woman's right to life and has not recognized the fetal rights. If a woman is competent and refuses medical treatment her decision must be respected even if fetus will suffer as a result. Fetus has no legal rights until it is born alive. A physician must respect the right of a competent pregnant woman patient to accept or reject any medical care recommended.

58. Induced abortion: Should not be used as an alternative to contraception. Counseling on contraception must be readily available—immediately. No delay in provision of abortion services. Physicians should not be compelled or discriminated or punished. Induced abortion should be uniformly available to all women in Canada and health care insurance should cover the costs.

59. Consent: Capable patients can refuse Rx. This decision must be respected even if it leads to serious harm or death. An incapable patient can be treated unless they refused treatment earlier when they were capable of self-determination.

60. Interactions with health care staff: Often while working a physician you have to maintain ethical and professional values and principles. There will be stations to test your way of interaction with your health care colleagues. Some of the examples are given below

a. Pharmacist not dispensing the OCP to your patient.
b. A physiotherapist becoming upset and agitated.

Section 11

Miscellaneous cases

Here is a list of cases from all sections that can appear in exams.

1. A 4 year old child presents with infrequent and hard bowel movements

Change in diet, toilet training, urinary incontinence, overflow incontinence
Enemas, medications, encopresis
Psychological factors
Problem solving: Hisrshsprung's disease, hypothyroidism, spinal bifida, anal fissures, diabetes mellitus, hypercalcemia, intestinal obstruction.
Manage: Increase fiber and water in diet, promote proper toilet training.

2. 12 year old female with leg pain

Pain questions.
Orthopedic history, collagen vascular diseases.
Look for normal growth and development.
Look for atropy, swelling, weaknesses, effusions.
Growing pain: does not occur in the joints—It occurs in the muscle area.
Perthes disease
Osgood Schlaters disease

3. *50 year old presents with left lower quadrant pain*

D/d Diverticulitis, tumor, IBD, hernia, in females: ectopic pregnancy, ovarian mass, cyst rupture, torsion of fibroid, PID, endometriosis, renal colic.
A per rectal examination is a must for all surgical stations. Usually, the SP/examiner will tell "noted, no need to do it/proceed"

4. *Patient coming with sore throat*

D/d: infectious mononucleosis (bilaterally enlarged posterior cervical nodes), A beta hemolytic streptococcal infection, viral (coughing, runny nose, hoarseness), dental problems, leukemia.

5. *40 year old C/o tinnitus*

Webber's and Rinne's test. Examine the ears. Conduct a full neurological exam.
M.S, tumours, acoustic neuroma, venous hums, labyrinthitis, Menier's disease.
Clanging or fluctuating tinnitus with visual hallucinations—think of temporal lobe epilepsy.
Drugs—salicylates, indomethacin, carbamazepine, L-dopa—all can cause tinnitus.
Order drug levels, consult ENT, and consult neurology.

6. *Motor vehicle accident followed by abdominal pain*

Diagnostic peritoneal lavage is positive if there is presence of gross blood, presence of bacteria, foreign material, RBC more than 100,000, WBCs more than 500.

7. *40 year old with bleeding per rectum*

Diverticular disease, angiodysplasia, ischemic colitis, ulcerative colitis, hemorrhoids, coagulation disorders, radiation injury, hereditary hemorrhagic telangiectasia, cancer, duodenal ulcer. Paediatrics (less than 1 year old)—intussuception, hemolytic uremic syndrome, Meckel's diverticulum.
Immediate management should be to stabilize the patient with IV fluids.
Radionuclear scanning/angiography to find out the source of bleeding.

8.   3 year old with wheezing

History of CF, weight loss, fever, atopy.
Rx with oxygen, nebulized salbutamol, atrovent, IV cortisol.
Use of puffers, supportive humidification.
Foreign body—bronchoscopy
Pneumonia—antibiotics and admit.

9.   20 year old male with polyuria, polydipsia. Take H/o and examine

progression, weight loss, fatigue, visual problems, SOB, diplopia, CNS palsies, hypertension, claudication, peripheral neuropathies, last insulin injection, family H/o, hyperlipidemia, medications, allergies, pancreatic surgeries, ethanol and illicit drug use.
Examine eyes, oral cavity, thyroid, CVS, ensure that the patient is stable.
Management: refer to a diabetic health center, refer to an endocrinologist, and maintain blood sugar levels, proper diet, and exercise. For diabetic ketoacidosis give 500cc of normal saline to correct the volume depletion; start insulin, monitor blood sugar, lytes, ABGs, search for a cause, possible infections etc.
Management is important before data collection to make sure that the patient is stable.

10.   2 year old child was brought by parents after having seizures

D/d: febrile seizures, absence seizures, trauma, child abuse (keep in mind), meningitis, Munchausen by proxy (rare)

11.   35 year old lady with a uterus that is large for date at 28 weeks

Confirm the LMP, maternal history, social history, drug abuse, history of diabetes, multiple pregnancies. Examine for lie and presentation.
If this is the first visit do CBC, cross and type blood, Rh antibody, rubella, VDRL, Pap smear, culture for Group B streptococci, chlamydia, HBS Ag, urine analysis for glucose and protein, blood pressure, blood glucose screen. Do ultrasound and biophysical profiles (NST's, fetal movement, fetal tone, fetal breathing, amniotic fluid volumes)
Fundal height is equal to gestational age from 22 weeks onwards.

If 2-3 cm more, then suggestive of multiple pregnancies. Also think of uterine difficulties, renal agenesis, molar pregnancies and choriocarcinoma.

12. A female patient with bilateral LN enlargement in the neck for the last 2 weeks. H/o viral infection, nasal stuffiness, discharge. O/E bilateral LN enlargement

D/d—inflammatory autoimmune disease (sarcoidosis, lupus), TB, liver disease with portal hypertension, painful LNs, painful bones, pruritis, wt. loss.
Family H/o sarcoid.
Diagnosis: Infectious mononucleosis.

13. Case: 68 year old Mr.X is concerned about his hearing

Examination: Examine for perception of spoken voice on both ears—check whether can hear whispering or sound of rubbing fingers.
Examine for cerumen, foreign body, tympanic membrane—perforation or sclerosis.
Weber test: look for lateralization
Rinne's test: Air and bone conduction
Examine heart, lungs and abdomen
D/d: Presbycusis, sensory motor hearing loss, familial hearing loss
D/w: Audiometry

14. A 30 yearl old pregnant woman fails to progress in labour

Causes include false labour, increased sedation, hyperactive or hypoactive contractions.
Arrest of active phase can be due to a large fetus, malpresentations, fetal anomaly, shoulder dystocia, abnormal shape of the pelvis.
Stages of labour. Latent phase—cervical effacement and dilatation up to 4 cm.
Active phase—cervical dilation to maximum size of 10 cm.
Second stage—delivery of the foetus.
Third stage—delivery of the placenta.

15. 23 year old female with a long history of long intervals of amenorrhea followed by prolonged vaginal bleeding

Pregnancy, polycystic ovarian disease, hypo or hyperthyroidism, prolactinomas, exercise induced, anorexia nervosa.
Primary or secondary amenorrhoea, outflow track problems.

Drug history, BCP, smoking and family history.
Beta HCG, prolactin level, TSH, estrogen levels, FSH/LH ratio.
Sexual history, previous attempts to have children.

16.   *An asymptomatic female presents with a mobile mass on pelvic exam*

Pain related to menstrual cycle.
GI or GU symptoms (diarrhoea, constipation, melena, rectal pain)
Vaginal bleeding, age at menarche, recent periods, pregnancy, contraception, history of PID, (abesses, hydrosalpings), history of leiomyoma, ovarian neoplasms, ectopic pregnancies, history of Crohn's disease.
Smoking, alcohol and trauma.
Physical exam for lymph nodes, chest, breasts and pelvic structures.
Abdominal and rectal/vaginal exam.
Investigations: X ray, CT, MRI, barium enema, IVP, beta HCG, alpha feto proteins, CA125 for ovarian carcinoma, CEA for metastatic colonic carcinoma, LFT and CBC.
Masses can be uterine or adnexal.
Non-ovarian masses can be ectopic pregnancies, appendicle or diverticular abesses
If during menstrual period and if mass is less than 8 cm, it is likely a functional cyst.

17.   *A 55 year old female with vulvuar discharge, pruritis, bleeding and irriations*

Is the lady post-menopausal? Has she ever had discharge before?
Recent antibiotics, yeast infections, sexual activity, new partners, contraception.
Condoms, pregnancy, STD's in the past. Frequency, dysuria and urgency.
Carcinoma, previous biopsies of the cervix or vulva.
Diabetes, Crohn's disease, Becets, cirrhosis and genital warts.
Herpes, family history of cancers. ROS.
Management: Biopsy (uterine and cervical)
CBC, lytes, BUN, hepatic function and creatinine.
Culture and sensitivity of the discharge.

18.   *22 year old female presents with actue right lower quadrant pain*

Stabilize the patient if needed.
Has this occurred before? Last meal, LMP, sexual activity.
PID, dysuria, pregnancy, jaundice.

Appendectomy, abdominal surgery, ovarian cyst, kidney stones.
Ethanol, trauma, IUD, infertility.
Per rectal examination.
Management: Nothing by mouth (NPO), CBC, differential, lytes, BUN, creatinine, amylase, beta HCG, PT, PTT.
Pelvic ultrasound, chest X ray.
D/d: appendicitis, cholecystitis, ectopic pregnancy, diverticulitis, pancreatitis, salpingitis, torsion ovary.

19. Vaginal bleed in a female aged 30 years

a. In a non-pregnant patient.
Reproductive age—hypothyroidism, DUB, Ca Cx, fibroid uterus, cervical polyp, cervicitis.
Menopausal—fibroid, Ca uterus, atopic vaginitis. Always do the ABC in any bleeding.
Blood dyscrasiasis, anticoagulant medication, family history of bleeding disorders.
Ask for any vaginal discharge. Number of partners, UTI symptoms, DM.
b.pregnant patient.
1. Less than 20 weeks of gestation—abortion (complete, incomplete, threatened)
2. More than 20 weeks of gestation—Placental previa (no pain), abruption placenta (pain)
Pain > bleeding—ectopic pregnancy.

20. Abdominal pain in a female aged 32 who is not pregnant

Acute—Gynecological—twisted ovarian cyst, PID, tuboovarian abscess, ectopic.
—Surgical—Acute appendicitis, renal colic, diverticulitis.
Chronic—chronic PID, endometriosis, adhesions, adenomyosis, interstitial cystitis, retroverted uterus, bladder stones

21. 30 year old with an unruptured ectopic pregnancy

Risk factors—PID, IUD, pelvic surgery, previous ectopics
Rx—conservative—if unruptured and beta HCG is < 10,000 and if size of sac is <3,5 cm
and if RFT,LFT and CBC are normal—Rx methotrexate. Give on day 1, 4, and 7
Success rate 90%.

22.   32 year old female with size larger than date with hyperemesis gravidarum

Vesicular mole is a possibility.
Asian, > 40 years, multiparity, hyperthyroidism, hypertension.

23.   31 week pregnant with pain and vaginal bleeding

Abruptio placenta.
Risk factors—previous abruptions, pre-eclampsia, age > 35 years, smoker, cocaine use, folate deficiency, polyhydramnios and rupture of membranes.

24.   20 year old lady wants to know about Pap smear

Tested from age 19 to 69
After 3 normal paps in 3 consecutive years, screening is needed every 2 years
If between 60-69 years old and if she had 4 normal Pap tests done, further screening may be discontinued.
Smear is taken close to the midcycle. Warm the spatula with warm water.
Do not use any lubricants. Use both spatula and brush
Spatula rotate 360 degrees
Brush rotate 90 degrees. Not used in pregnancy.
Both the samples are smeared parallel to each other on a glass slide
Fix it immediately. Dry and mail it.
If positive—colposcopy. If ca in situ—cone biopsy.

25.   32 year old lady diagnosed with endometriosis

Nulliparous, Age 25-45, positive family history.
Short cycles and long menstrual period.
Eg. every 20 days and lasting for 7-8 days.
Mild abdominal pain during periods.
Weakness.

26.   25 year old with vaginal discharge and knee joint pain. Has a new partner

Gonococcal infection.
Gonococcal arthritis.
Take swabs from cervix, rectum, urethra, pharynx and skin.
Inform public health.
Rx the partner.

27. 40 years old woman comes to your office complaining of heartburn

OCD: How long? All the time? Special timing?

After meals? Is it getting worse? Just heartburn or also other symptoms?

Determine: If pain (PQRST), position that relieve/aggravate, meds, food (fat, chocolate, tomato, gas beverages).

Associated symptoms: Stomach ache, N/V, wheezing, bringing up acid, cough, hoarseness, dysphagia, bloating, belching, melena, fullness, CP, SOB, palpitations, ear pain.

PMH: PUD, CAD, asthma, esophageal hernia/procedures, anemia, GI cancer.

Medications: ASA, NSAIDS, BCP, Vit C, Iron, BP Medications, Tums (antacid).

Smoking, alcohol, drugs, coffee, dietary habits, occupation, stress, weight (obesity).

Family H/o (GI cancer).

Case: GERD

28. Elderly man with Cr 1000. Take H/o. Give DDx. What investigations would you order?

Prerenal: Hypovolemia, septicaemia, cardiac failure, liver failure.

Post renal (obstructive): Prostatism, tumour, stones.

Renal: Acute tubular injury due to renal toxins, ischemia, X-ray contrast, myoglobinuria, acute glomerulonephritis, DIC, pyelonephritis, intrarenal precipitation in hypercalcemia and myeloma.

Investigations: CBC, lytes, BUN, Cr, PO_4, Ca^{++}, Mg, INR/PTT, AST, ALT, Alk. Phos., GGT, PSA, CK-MB, ABG, Urinalysis: microscopy, C&S, abdominal X-ray, abdominal-pelvic U/S, post-void catheterization (Avoid IVP due to dye problems).

29. Female patient found to have a nodule on routine CXR. Perform a focussed P/E. Give a DDx. What investigations would you order?

Granuloma (scar tissue from old pneumonia, TB granuloma, histoplasmosis, silicosis, sarcoid), tumour (benign or malignant), lung abscess, AV malformation.

Investigations: Old chest X-ray for comparison (if lesion is old and unchanging, interventions are less aggressive), CT chest (helical) with CT guided needle biopsy, sputum for cytology and acid-fast staining (TB), TB skin test, bronchoscopy with biopsy and washings if lesion seen.

30.   A 25 yearl old female with migratory type of arthritis for the last 2 weeks

Migratory arthritis suggests gonococcal infection
Onset of arthritic symptoms, durations, joints affected and chronology.
Associated fever, malaise, fatigue, rash, abdominal pain and cramps, vaginal discharge, pain with urination, dyspareunia.
H/o of arthritis (rheumatoid, osteoarthritis), psoriasis, Lyme disease (travel to Southern Ontario, camping trips), Reiter's syndrome, ankylosing spondylitis.
STDs including PID. Sexual H/o: present partners, number of partners, fidelity of partner(s), and use of condoms.
Medications, drugs, alcohol, smoking, allergies, PMH, family H/o, ROS.
DDx: Gonococcal arthritis, psoriatic arthritis, Lyme disease, Reiter's syndrome, ankylosing spondylitis, rheumatoid arthritis, osteoarthritis, gout.
Investigations: CBC, ESR, lytes, urea, Cr, INR, PTT, blood cultures. Cervical swab for culture and sensitivity. Joint aspirate for microscopy and culture.

31.   Assess the volume status of a patient

Look for both body fluid deficiency and excess.
Head—Eyes, moist mouth, wet arm pits?
Neck—JVP measure, hepatojugular reflex (press for 30 sec)
Base of the lung—Auscultate—fluid (left sided heart failure)
Heart—S3, S4 for gallop rhythm
Abdomen for ascitis
Hepatomegaly, splenomegaly (right sided heart failure)
Legs—Pitting edema
Skin turger
Peripheral pulse—Volume and rate
Capillary refill
Sacral edema

32.   Patient kicked by a horse, now hypotensive in ER. Manage

Resuscitation.
Check for abnormalities on abdominal exam suggestive of splenic rupture.
With clear surgical abdomen (rigidity, rebound, absence of bowel sounds), consult general surgery and prepare patient for immediate OR.
If less severe abdominal bleeding is suspected, consider CT abdomen or diagnostic peritoneal lavage.

33. Patient with very severe asthma. O/E—O_2 sat <90%; FEV1<40%)

Intubate.
100% oxygen
Salbutamol 4-8 puffs by MDI q 20 min x 3 times or by nebulizer 5 mg q20 min x 3 times.
Anticholinergics (Ipatropium) 4-8 puffs q 20 min x 3 or by nebulizer 0.25 mgm q20 min x 3 times.
Methyl prednisolone—125 mgm IV or hydrocortisone 500 mg I.V.

34. Anaphylactic reaction in ER manage

ABCs secure.
On scene epi-pen.
Moderate signs: 0.5ml of 1:1000 solution of epinephrine IM.
Severe signs: 1 ml of 1:1000 solution of epinephrine by ETT or IV.
Cardiac monitoring.
Diphenhydramine 50 mgm IM or IV every 4-6 hrs.
Mehyl prednisolone-50 to 100 mgm IV.
Salbutamol—via nebulizer/glucagon (for those who are on beta blockers)—10 microgm every 1 min IV.

35. 60 yr old man with microscopic hematuria on routine analysis. Take H/o. Give DDx. What investigations would be helpful?

Has the patient noticed any gross hematuria.
UTI symptoms: Dysuria, frequency, urgency, fever, nausea and vomiting.
Malignancy symptoms: Decreased appetite and weight loss, night sweats.
Obstructive symptoms: Difficulty initiating stream, poor flow, dribbling.
Pain in the abdomen, back, groin or loins.
PMH: Malignancy, kidney stones, UTI, prostate disease.
Medications, Allergies, family H/o, ROS.
DDx: Renal cancer, bladder cancer, renal calculi, glomerulonephritis, UTI.
Investigations: Urine for microscopy, culture and sensitivity; abdominal-pelvic u/s; cystoscopy, intravenous contrast urography, IVP.

36. 62 yr old man presents to the ER department with 12 hr suprapubic discomfort and inability to urinate. Catheterization yields 1200 cc urine. Take H/o. What is the most likely cause of this man's problem? Give three other possible diagnoses. What tests will you order?

H/o of suprapubic pain and inability to urinate.

H/o of pain on urination, frank blood in the urine, colour of urine, difficulty initiating or maintaining stream, fever, renal pain, groin pain.

Previous renal colic/prostate hypertrophy, prostate cancer, prostatism, nephrolithiasis?

Malignant symptoms: Night sweats, weight loss, fatigue.

Medications, drugs/alcohol, smoking, past medical H/o,

Past surgical H/o, H/o of pelvic radiation, TURP, family H/o, review of systems.

Most likely diagnosis: Benign prostatic hyperplasia.

D/d: UTI, prostatitis, prostate cancer.

Investigations: Urea/creatinine, urinalysis, PSA, renal ultrasound.

38. *Small for gestational age*

Maternal—Nutritional intake, smoking, drug abuse, ethanol abuse.

Placental—Intrapartum hemorrhage, Torch infections.

Foetal—cyanotic heart disease, pulmonary insufficiency, hypertension, chronic renal disease.

IUGR—when birth weight is less than the 10th percentile for their gestational age.

APGAR—score is calculated from heart rate, respiratory rate, muscle tone, body color, and responsiveness.

39. *Breast self exam*

Sitting: Palpation of axillary, infraclavicular and supraclavicular nodes.

Inspect breasts with hands above head and pressing fists on hips.

Inspect for dimpling, nipple retraction, peau d'orange around nipple.

Supine (with pillow under shoulder): Rotatory palpation of 4 quadrants and nipple squeeze.

Can denote position of lumps by clock position with cm distance from nipple.

Watch for bloody nipple discharge and inflammation.

Yearly mammography screening of proven benefit from age 50. Benefit as a screening test equivocal for age 40 in the general population but is recommended if there is a positive family H/o of breast cancer.

Breast cancer in two first degree relatives (parents, siblings, and children) is an indication for yearly mammography starting at 5-10 yrs before youngest family member's presentation.

40. Mother with low birth weight baby, just delivered. Take H/o. On P/E of the baby you find emaciation with wrinkled yellow skin and yellow tears. What is the problem? Give 3 underlying causes for this. Give 2 potential problems, which may arise in the next 48 hrs.

IUGR:

a.   Symmetric (normal head to body size): Familial, gestational infections (ToRCH) toxoplasmosis (carried in cat faeces), rubella, CMV, herpes.
b.   Asymmetric (small body): Placental insufficiency due to maternal malnutrition, smoking, drugs and alcohol, illness during pregnancy, hypertension.
Jaundiced, emaciated body: ABO or Rh incompatibility, neonatal liver insufficiency (CMV), and sepsis (ToRCH)
Two potential problems arising in the next 48 hrs:
f.   Kernicterus (hyperbilirubinemic seizures and brain damage)
g.   Hydrops faetalis (generalized and pulmonary edema, with high output heart failure).

41. 58 yr old woman in hospital 4 days post-op hysterectomy for fibroids. Agitated, had tactile hallucinations the previous night. Take H/o. Finding: H/o of alcoholism. What is the most likely diagnosis?

Onset of hallucinations, duration, description.
Tactile hallucinations or bugs crawling on skin or on ceiling suggest alcohol withdrawal.
Associated fever, agitation, sweating, tremor, decreased consciousness, seizure?
Any problems with surgical recovery, wound healing, mobilization?
Amount of alcohol consumed at home. H/o of alcoholism?
Post-op medications (morphine, demerol (meperidine, is an opioid analgesic). Previous bad reactions to these or to antibiotics?
Previous episode like this one? PMH, medications, drug and alcohol abuse, smoking, allergy, family H/o, ROS.
Most likely Dx: Alcohol withdrawal.

42. Young man with a swollen cervical lymph node. Perform a focussed P/E.
Case2. CXR shows mediastinal widening with perihilar nodes. Describe. Give 5 features on H/o which would be helpful for diagnosis?

Abdominal Exam: Palpate for lymph nodes in the neck, supra and infra-clavicular, axillae, groin.
Examine the oral cavity and pharynx.

Check for rashes.

DDx: Lymphoma, leukemia, viral infection (mononucleosis, HIV, EBV), inflammatory autoimmune disease (sarcoidosis, lupus), serum sickness (severe allergic reaction short of anaphylaxis), TB, liver disease with portal hypertension.

Five features on H/o helpful for Dx: Viral prodrome, family H/o of sarcoid, lymph nodes painful, bone pain, pruritis, weight loss.

43. A young man sustains a head injury on falling from his bicycle. Patient has been hemodynamically stabilized. Perform a focussed neurological exam. Lateral skull and lateral C-spine X-rays provided. Are they normal? The patient has continuing sanguineous discharge from his nose. What is the likely cause of this? What is the treatment?

Continuous sanguineous nasal discharge after head injury is likely a leak of CSF mixed with blood. This is due to injury of the meninges and can in less than 5% of cases lead to meningitis.

Prophylactic antibiotics are not indicated as this breeds resistant organisms.

If meningitis results, it is usually due to less virulent organisms than in other settings. >90% of leaks resolve spontaneously within 4 weeks.

If leak does not spontaneously resolve, surgical repair may be necessary.

Consult neurosurgery.

44. Older man with 55 RBC/hpf on routine urinalysis. Take a focussed H/o. What is the likely diagnosis? Give differential diagnoses. What 2 investigations would you order?

Suprapubic pain, pain on urination, frequency, urgency, frank blood in the urine (globular clots from bladder or string-shaped clots from ureters), colour of urine, difficulty initiating or maintaining urinary stream, renal pain, groin pain.

Fever, chills, nausea, fatigue. Previous renal colic/diagnosed nephrolithiasis?

H/o of hypercalcemia, hypertension.

Malignant symptoms: Night sweats, weight loss, fatigue.

Medications, drugs/alcohol, smoking, anticoagulants and salicylates

PMH, past surgical H/o, family H/o (polycystic kidney disease), ROS.

Likely Dx: Benign prostatic hypertrophy

DDx: Nephrolithiasis, hydronephrosis, UTI, prostatitis, prostate cancer, transitional cell carcinoma of the bladder, renal cell carcinoma, essential hematuria (tends to occur in children).

Investigations: PSA, IVP, renal and prostate U/S

45. *Young female with malaise, tender lymph nodes in the neck, LUQ abdominal pain. Perform a focussed P/E. Give DDx.*

Abdominal exam: Palpate for lymph nodes in the neck, supra and infra-clavicular, axillae, groin.
Examine the oral cavity and pharynx. Check for rashes.
Neoplastic: Lymphoma, leukemia.
Viral: Mononucleosis, HIV, EBV.
Bacterial: Syphilis.
Inflammatory autoimmune disease: Sarcoidosis, lupus.
Liver disease with portal hypertension. Serum sickness, allergic reaction.

46. *Case: 37 year old Mrs. X wants to know more about Down's syndrome. Talk to he.*

A baby with Down's syndrome can be born to any couple.
However risk increases with increasing maternal age.
Normal population 1/800; Maternal age 35-39 1/300; Maternal age 40-45 1/80
Some Down's syndrome person can have productive lives; but many have physical and mental disabilities.
Usually life span is short. No way to predict how serious the disability will be.
No cure for Down's syndrome. Relatives have nearly an 8% increased chance.
Early diagnosis is important to decide for the future of the pregnancy.
16-18 weeks by amniocentesis: AFP (alpha feto protein) decreases in Down's syndrome.
Fine needle is put into the abdomen. Some cramping and spotting for 1-2 days is normal. If father is Rh +ive and mother Rh-ive- need to administer Rhogam in 1-2 days.
If abnormal results occur, refer to a genetic counselor.
Risk of amniocentesis for a miscarriage: Normal risk at 16-18 weeks is 3.5%. Amniocentesis will increase the risk by 1%. So the total risk is 4.5%.

47. *Case: Mrs. X is a 32 years old woman who is going to give birth to her baby next month. She wants to know more about the delivery procedure. Talk to her.*

Prenatal classes: lectures, regular labor room visits, get introduced to the birthing team, Lamaze classes.
On the labor day: Give partner—family support, experienced nursing assistance, relaxed controlled breathing technique, confortable labor position, can walk around in between contractions, What would you like for pain? Massage, Jacuzzi, hot bath.

Analgesics: IM Demerol (meperidine) 50 mgm IM (Check for foetal heart)

Anaesthesia: Inhalation NO; Self medication; Local: lidocaine; Regional: Epidural anaesthesia-when cervix is 4 cm dilated; given by an anaesthetist; sign a consent form;

Is done by putting a fine needle in the back and continue to monitor BP.

Episiotomy increase chances of dysparenuria; There fore, without it tear comes and suture it. Tear heals better.

Section 12

Physical Examination

- <u>Rule No:1</u> Read the question carefully. If asked for P/Examination, never take H/o.
- <u>Rule No:2</u> If it is H/o and P/E, stop H/o by midway. Then conduct the physical.
- P/Examination is same as standard P/Examination books.
- The major differences and points to remember are the following.
- Always cover the areas that you are not examining.
- Ask patient to move the sheet little down
- Put the sheet back after the examination
- Tell the patient what you are going to do.
- Also tell the patient to tell you if it hurts.
- For abdominal examination the order is Inspection, Auscultation, Palpation and Percussion.
- Take measurements whenever it is needed.
- Tell about opthalmoscopic exam (you don't need to do it; but tell).
- Do a per rectal exam in all surgical cases (you don't need to do it; but tell).
- Time will run very fast. Adjust your time during P/Examination.
- Thank the patient.

Section 13

A sample station

Case: Female patient with vaginal discharge and mild fever. Take history

- Read the questions well. Try to memorize the name of the patient.
- Think of 5 D/d and mentally prepare for questions pertaining to all of them.
- See how many tasks you are asked to do. If there is H/o and P/E, divide your time 50%:50%
- Wish the patient by name, shake hands and introduce yourself (Firm with ladies as well!!!)
- Keep a reasonable distance from the patient while you sit or stand.
- Starting words may be—"I am here to talk to your regarding your problem" Can you tell more about it?
- Sensitive issues "Talk in a confidential way" I will keep it a confidential one"
- Let patient talk—Don't interrupt (first question—open ended).Ask about vaginal discharge. Take complete history.........(Not explained here).
- For P/Es, make the patient comfortable. Tell them what you are going to do. "This examination might cause some pain. Let me know if you feel any pain".
- Don't undress the patient. Ask the patient to do it for you. Also ask whether you want to leave the room while patient undress.

- Always draw a sheet up before the patient pulls her gown up.
- If the patient is showing pain, tell that you will give enough pain killers once the examination is over. Be empathetic.
- When you hear the 8th minute bell (in a 10 minute station)—do EPP2Q Explain, Prognosis, Plan/2Quesitons
- Explain what the patient is suffering from.
- "I believe that you are suffering from a disease called pelvic inflammatory disease. Usually it is caused by sexually transmitted diseases. We are going to do a Pap smear and some blood tests. Whatever we have talked today will be confidential".
- "Your partner/husband also need treatment at this point, as he is likely to be infected".
- If patient says "no", tell that the positive result will automatically be reported from the laboratory and a social worker will approach you and your partner after a few days.
- Also I would like to inform you that once the lab reports are ready, I may have to inform the public health if it turn out to be Chlamydia, Gonorrhea, Syphilis (Not for herpes simplex and papiloma virus).
- I need your consent to call your husband/partner for discussion and treatment (in case of STDs).
- Is this treatment plan work for you?
- Tell the prognosis e.g. "Mrs. X, you are going to be alright."/"Mrs.X, You need to stay in the hospital for a few days"/"Mrs.X, you require an emergency surgery" etc.
- Tell the plan. e.g. "I am going to prescribe you some medications. This medication will take 3 weeks to show the effects. We will meet again after 3 weeks". In the mean time if you have any serious problems, please contact us for arranging a visit".
- Always involve the patient in decision making. If there are more than 1 treatment options, inform the patient and if necessary help him/her to chose one (especially between surgical/medical management
- Thank the patient.

Section 14

Examination Formats—U.S and Canadian

U.S

- The test has 10-12 stations (1 or 2 may be experimental stations. You will not know which those stations are and they will not be counted for evaluation).
- Each station is called Integrated Clinical Encounter (ICE) and has 2 parts
  a. Data gathering for 15 minutes—history taking and physical examination.
  b. Patient note writing for 10 minutes.
- Therefore, your written English needs to be improved. Write legibly. If your hand writing needs improvement, practice writing skills.
- Organize your time appropriately. i. e. 7.5 minutes for history taking and 7.5 minutes for physical examination.

Canada

A. OSCE by different provinces (Ontario, Alberta, Mannitoba, British Columbia)

- Usually consist of 14 stations of which 2 will not be counted for scoring
- All of them will be of same duration i.e. 10 minutes each with a break after 7 stations.
- Usually 2 stations will be ethical situations to solve.

B.   MCCQE part 2

- Usually 14 stations of which 2 will not be counted for scoring.
- 8 of them will be long stations of 10 minutes each. 6 of them will be short stations of 5 minute duration followed by 5 minutes to write answers to questions, including X-rays, EKGs, growth charts, KUB, blood and urine results etc.

Abbreviations

#—Fracture
AA—Alcoholics anonymous
AAA—Abdominal aortic aneurysm
AB—Antibiotics
ABG—Arterial blood gases
AF—Atrial fibrillation\
AIDS—Acquired immune deficiency syndrome
aPTT—Activated partial thromboplastin time
ASA—Acetyl salicylic acid
BBT—Basal body temperature
BCP—Birth control pills
BD/BID-Two times a day
BPV—Benign positional vertigo
BM—Bowel movements
BMI—Body mass index
BP—Blood pressure
BUN—Blood urea nitrogen
Ca—Cancer
CABG—Coronary artery bypass grafting
CAD—Coronary artery disease
CAS—Children's aid society
CBC—Complete blood count
CCU—Cardiac care unit
CF—Cystic fibrosis
CHF—Congestive heart failure
C/o—Complaining of
COPD—Chronic obstructive pulmonary disease
CP—Cerebral palsy/Chest pain/Costo-phrenic
CPAP—Continuous positive airway pressure
CPR—Cardiopulmonary resuscitation
CS—Caesarian section
CT—Computed tomography
CTD—Connective tissue disease
CVA—Cerebro-vascular accident
CVP—Central venous pressure

Cx—Cervix
CXR—Chest X-ray
D/c—Discharge
D/d—DDx
DDx—DDx
DRE—Digital rectal exam
DDx—DDx
DH—Dehydration
DNR—Do not resuscitate
DM—Diabètes mellites
DRE—Digital rectal examination
DTR—Deep tendon reflexes
DVT—Deep venous thrombosis
DWU—Diagnostic workup
Dx—Diagnosis
ECASA—Enteric coated acetyl salicylic acid
ECG—Electrocardiogram
EEG—Electroencephalogram
EKG—Electrocardiogram
ED—Emergency department
EDC—Expected date of confinement
ENT—Ear, nose, throat
EOM—Extraoccular muscles
ER—Emergency room
EtOH—Alcohol
Ext.—Extremities
FD—Family doctor
FH—Family history
F/Vs—Follow up
FTT—Failure to thrive
F/U—Follow up
GAD—Generalized anxiety disorder
GB—Gall bladder
GCS—Glasgow coma scale
GER—Gastro-esophageal reflux
GI—Gastro-intestinal
GTPAL—Gravida/Para/Pregnancies/Abortions/Living
GU—Genitourinary
HEENT—Head, eyes, ears, nose, throat
HIV—Human immunodeficiency virus

H/o—History of
HPV—Human papilloma virus
HR—Heart rate
HRT—Hormone replacement therapy
HTN—hypertension
H/o—History
ILD—Inflammatory lung disease
IBD—Inflammatory bowel disease
IDDM—Insulin dependent diabetes mellitus
IM—Intramuscularly
INR—International normalized ratio
IUGR—Intrauterine growth retardation
IV—Intravenously
JVD—Jugular venous distention
JVP—Jugular venous pulsation
K—Potassium
KUB—Kidney, ureter, bladder
L—Left
LMP—Last menstrual period
LOC—Loss of consciousness
LOV—Loss of vision
LN—Lymph node
LP—Lumbar puncture
MDD—Maniac depressive disorder
MEN—Multiple endocrine neoplasia
MI—Myocardial Infarction
MOT—Ministry of Transportation
MMSE—Mini mental status examination
MR—Mental retardation
MRI—Magnetic resonance imaging
MS—Multiple sclerosis
MSK—Musculoskeletal system
MVA—Motor vehicle accident'
Mx—Management
NKA—No known allergies
NKDA—No known drug allergies
NL—Normal limits
NPO-Nothing by mouth
NS—Normal saline
NSR—Normal sinus rhythm

N/V—Nausea and vomiting
NIDDM—Non-insulin dependent diabetes mellites
OA—Osteoarthritis
OCD—Onset, course, duration/Obsessive compulsive disorder
OCP—Oral contraceptive pills
OGD—Oesophago-gastric disease
OM—Otitis Media
OPD—Out patient department
OR—Operation room
O—Bottle
P—Pulse
PA—Postero-anterior
PCD—Polycystic ovarian disease
PCOD—Polycystic ovarian disease
P/E—Physical examination
PEARL—Pupil equal and reacting to light
PERLA—Pupil equal, react to light and accommodation
PFT—Pulmonary function test
PID—Pelvic inflammatory bowel disease
PMH—Past medical H/o
PMS—Post-menopausal symptoms
PND—Paroxysmal nocturnal dyspnoea
PO—By mouth
PQRST—Pointation, Quantity, Radiation, Severity, Transmission
PRBC—Packed RBCs
PROM—Premature rupture of membranes
PSA—Prostate specific antigen
PT—Prothrombin time
PTT—Partial prothrombin time
PUD—Peptic ulcer disease
q—Every
R—Right
RA—Rheumatoid arthritis
RAP—Recurrent abdominal pain
RBC—Red blood cells
RF—Risk factors/Renal failure
R/o—Rule out
ROS—Review of symptoms
RR—Respiratory rate
RUQ—Right upper quadrant

Rx—Treatment
SAH—Subarachnoid hemorrhage
SB—Short bowel
SH—Social history
SOB—Shortness of breath
SP—Standardized patient
STD—Sexually transmitted disease
SAH—Subarachnoid hemorrhage
SVC—Superior vena cava
Sx—Surgery
T—Temperature
TCA—Tricyclic antidepressants
TIA—Transient ischemic attack
TURP—Transurethral resection of prostate
U/A—Urine analysis
URI—Upper respiratory tract infection
URTI—Upper respiratory tract infection
U/S—Ultrasound
USG—Ultrasonogram
UTI—Urinary tract infection
V/A—Visual acuity
WBC—White blood cells
WNL—Within normal limits
W/o—Without

978-0-595-39756-3
0-595-39756-5